LIVING WITH HUNTINGTON'S DISEASE

CHALLENGES, PERSPECTIVES AND QUALITY OF LIFE

SHERMAN HOWELL

EDITOR

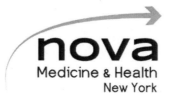

nova
Medicine & Health
New York

NOTICE TO THE READER

Library of Congress Cataloging-in-Publication Data

ISBN: 978-1-53616-729-0

Published by Nova Science Publishers, Inc. † New York

CONTENTS

PREFACE

Living with Huntington's Disease: Challenges, Perspectives and Quality of Life first discusses the variety of sleep disorders in Huntington's Disease, as well as how sleep quality can be associated with other important clinical symptoms.

Although Huntington's disease is categorized as a movement disorder, the wide range of non-motor symptoms including cognitive impairment and behavioral abnormalities are considered by patients and their caregivers to be just as disabling as the motor symptoms. As such, the authors explore the importance of symptomatic treatment of Huntington's disease-related symptoms.

Following this, the emotional and communicational issues in Huntington's disease and their interrelations are examined, including depressive symptomatology, anxiety, helplessness or anger, as well as verbal and non-verbal communication and assistive technology.

Lastly, the authors describe current trends and efforts in gene therapy techniques and the improvements in health conditions of Huntington's disease patients and their families.

Chapter 1 - The clinical onset of HD has historically been defined as the point when a person who carries a CAG-expanded HTT allele develops "the unequivocal presence of an otherwise unexplained extrapyramidal movement disorder" (for example, chorea, dystonia, slowing of saccade initiation and velocity). While the presence of motor symptoms is required for the clinical diagnosis of HD, the disease classically manifests with a triad of signs and symptoms, including not only motor but also cognitive and behavioral features. Psychiatric symptoms can be present across all stages of HD, even preceding the onset of motor impairment. Although not universal, they are common and may be a cause of significant distress in HD. Disturbed sleep is also a prominent feature of HD, substantially impairing the quality of life of both patients and their caregivers. By using polysomnography and actigraphy, studies have reported an increased sleep onset latency, sleep fragmentation and frequent nocturnal awakenings, reduced sleep efficiency, delayed and shortened rapid eye movement (REM) sleep, increased periodic leg movements, as well as circadian rhythm disturbances in patients with HD. However, sleep dysfunction in HD is likely to be underdiagnosed by clinicians and underreported by patients. Self-report of sleep problems in HD might be reduced because patients with HD may not present with excessive daytime sleepiness or do not report it, mainly due to their lack of insight into their symptoms. Nevertheless, when asked directly about the quality of their sleep, up to 90% of patients acknowledge having sleep problems. The vast majority of patients (~60%) rated sleep difficulties as either "very important" or "moderately important" components of the patient's overall health problems. Notwithstanding the high prevalence and the availability of clinical tools, sleep disorders are not routinely evaluated in patients with HD. Sleep disturbances can seriously affect the quality of life of the patient, caregiver, and family. In addition, sleep dysfunction can result in cognitive impairment, inattentiveness, poor memory, mood disorders and an increased risk of accidents and institutionalization. Identifying abnormalities in sleep patterns could significantly impact the management of patients with HD. This chapter intends to discuss the variety of sleep disorders in HD, as well as how sleep quality can be associated with other important clinical symptoms. Finally, the authors will comment on how HD treatment is associated with sleep disruption and present the therapeutic options for alleviating sleep problems in HD.

Chapter 2- Although HD is categorized as a movement disorder, the wide range of non-motor symptoms including cognitive impairment and behavioral abnormalities are considered by patients and their caregivers to be just as disabling as the motor symptoms. Motor and nonmotor symptomatic treatment is an important consideration to improve both functionality and quality of life in HD. A variety of symptomatic treatments are currently available. Pharmacological options for the motor symptoms include tetrabenazine and deutetrabenazine – the only two FDA-approved drugs for HD related chorea, neuroleptics, gabaergic and antiglutaminergic medications are often used off label. Antidepressants and neuroleptics are also used to treat the neuropsychiatiric symptoms. Interdisciplinary, non-pharmacological options are available such as, psychotherapy, physical, occupational and speech therapy, genetic counseling, social work and nutritional services. However, there is currently no approved disease-modifying therapy for HD. After the discovery of the genetic cause for HD 26 years ago, great efforts have been made to identify a treatment capable of modifying the disease course. Recent advances in therapeutic strategies promise an exciting era for clinical trials in HD. Increased recognition of the phenotypic variability in HD can also improve the symptomatic treatment goals. This endeavor will be coupled with advances in novel therapeutics, including strategies in lowering the mutant huntingtin protein and targeting the *HTT* gene. Future novel HD treatments are focused on positively impacting both quality of life and longevity in individuals with HD,, in addition to contributing to research in other neurodegenerative disorders. This chapter will present the past, current and future clinical trials targeting both symptomatic and disease-modifying treatments for HD.

Chapter 3 - Huntington's disease is a devastating neurological disorder impacting all aspects of individual functioning, including cognition, mood, self-care, social interaction and the capacity for work. Similarly to other patients with neurodegenerative diseases, Huntington sufferers face innumerable problems in everyday life, both within their bodies and psyches, and in the natural and social environments. The following chapter centers on emotional and communicational issues in Huntington's disease and their interrelations, covering a range of topics from depressive symptomatology, anxiety, helplessness or anger, to verbal and non-verbal communication and assistive technology. As the communication processes get increasingly disrupted during disease progression, knowing what the patient feels and needs represents a major challenge for both professional and lay caregivers. Simultaneously, the emotional stratum of a Huntington patient's personality is subject to various independent detrimental effects unrelated to communication. An overview of current research combined with personal stories is provided in the present chapter along with discussion of emotional suffering of all persons involved.

Chapter 4 - Huntington's disease (HD) is a genitive inheritance pathology disease that causes pleiotropic symptoms, including motor, cognitive, and psychiatric impairments. Mutations in the HTT gene (Ch.4 p. 16.3) cause the expansion of the CAG trinucleotide repeat region of the HTT gene, generating a long abnormal version of the huntingtin (HTT) protein. Moreover, the cell machinery forms small protein aggregates that accumulate in neurons, disrupting the normal cell functions. Current HD clinical treatments focus on attenuating symptoms with conventional therapies and pharmacological treatments, with limited effectiveness. Under those circumstances, current research aims to find new targets to promote the reduction of HD severity in patients. Recent evidence suggests that several neural functions regulated by epigenetic imprinting are disrupted in HD patients, resulting in the typical portrait of HD neuronal disorders. For instance, clinical and pre-clinical data of the epigenetic processes in HD indicate alterations in its regulatory pathways. In fact, epigenetic abnormalities namely, DNA methylation, post-translational modifications in nucleosome histones and biogenesis of the miRNA are dysregulated in HD´s experimental models and HD patients. Moreover, recent developments silencing HTT RNA messenger molecules through Antisense Oligonucleotides and its posterior degradation via RNase H1 enzyme have shown a significant reduction on mutant HTT protein expression in HD patients. These findings and recent research advances have set new research horizons to therapeutic targets and the establishment of more effective clinical treatments. Therefore, this chapter describes current trends and efforts in gene therapy techniques, and the improvements in health conditions of HD patients and their families.

In: Living with Huntington's Disease ISBN: 978-1-53616-729-0
Editor: Sherman Howell © 2020 Nova Science Publishers, Inc.

Chapter 1

SLEEP PROBLEMS IN HD

Natalia P. Rocha[1,2], PhD, Will K. Tanigaki[4],
Maria A. Rossetti[2,3], PhD, Sudha S. Tallavajhula[4,5], MD
and Erin Furr Stimming[2,4], MD

[1]Mitchell Center for Alzheimer's disease
and Related Brain Disorders, Department of Neurology,
The University of Texas Health Science Center, Houston, TX, US
[2]HDSA Center of Excellence at University
of Texas Health Science Center at Houston, Houston, TX, US
[3]Neurocognitive Disorders Center, Department of Neurology,
The University of Texas Health Science Center at Houston,
Houston, TX, US
[4]Department of Neurology,
The University of Texas Health Science Center, Houston, TX, US
[5]TIRR Memorial Hermann Neurological Sleep Disorders Center,
Houston, TX, US

ABSTRACT

The clinical onset of HD has historically been defined as the point when a person who carries a CAG-expanded HTT allele develops "the unequivocal presence of an otherwise unexplained extrapyramidal movement disorder" (for example, chorea, dystonia, slowing of saccade initiation and velocity). While the presence of motor symptoms is required for the clinical diagnosis of HD, the disease classically manifests with a triad of signs and symptoms, including not only motor but also cognitive and behavioral features. Psychiatric symptoms can be present across all stages of HD, even preceding the onset of motor impairment. Although not universal, they are common and may be a cause of significant distress in HD. Disturbed sleep is also a prominent feature of HD, substantially impairing the quality of life of both patients and their caregivers. By using polysomnography and actigraphy, studies have reported an increased sleep onset latency, sleep fragmentation and frequent nocturnal awakenings, reduced sleep efficiency, delayed and shortened rapid eye movement (REM) sleep, increased periodic leg movements, as well as circadian rhythm disturbances in patients with HD. However, sleep dysfunction in HD is likely to be underdiagnosed by clinicians and underreported by patients. Self-report of sleep problems in HD might be reduced because patients with HD may not present with excessive daytime sleepiness or do not report it, mainly due to their lack of insight into their symptoms. Nevertheless, when asked directly about the quality of their sleep, up to 90% of patients acknowledge having sleep problems. The vast majority of patients (~60%) rated sleep difficulties as either "very important" or "moderately important" components of the patient's overall health problems. Notwithstanding the high prevalence and the availability of clinical tools, sleep disorders are not routinely evaluated in patients with HD. Sleep disturbances can seriously affect the quality of life of the patient, caregiver, and family. In addition, sleep dysfunction can result in cognitive impairment, inattentiveness, poor memory, mood disorders and an increased risk of accidents and institutionalization. Identifying abnormalities in sleep patterns could significantly impact the management of patients with HD. This chapter intends to discuss the variety of sleep disorders in HD, as well as how sleep quality can be associated with other important clinical symptoms. Finally, we will comment on how HD treatment is associated with sleep disruption and present the therapeutic options for alleviating sleep problems in HD.

INTRODUCTION

Huntington's disease (HD) is a monogenic progressive neurodegenerative condition caused by a CAG repeat expansion in the huntingtin (*HTT*) gene on chromosome 4 that codes for polyglutamine in the huntingtin protein (HTT) (Ross et al. 2014). The pathognomonic pathological signature of HD consists of intranuclear inclusion bodies, which are large aggregates of abnormal HTT in neuronal nuclei. Aggregates also arise elsewhere in the cell, including the cytoplasm, dendrites, and axon terminals (Ross and Tabrizi 2011). Neuropathological abnormalities in HD develop well before evident symptoms, are progressive, and eventually involve the entire brain, resulting in about 25% brain weight loss in advanced HD. Nonetheless, the most prominent neuropathology in HD occurs within the striatal part of the basal ganglia, in which gross atrophy is accompanied by extensive neuronal loss and astrogliosis (Reiner, Dragatsis, and Dietrich 2011).

The clinical onset of HD is defined as the point when a person who carries a CAG-expanded HTT allele develops "the unequivocal presence of an otherwise unexplained extrapyramidal movement disorder" (for example, chorea, dystonia, slowing of saccades, bradykinesia, rigidity) (Ross et al. 2014). While the presence of motor symptoms is required for the clinical diagnosis of HD, the disease classically manifests with a triad of signs and symptoms, including not only motor but also cognitive and behavioral features (Duff et al. 2010; Epping et al. 2016). Psychiatric symptoms can be present across all stages of HD, even preceding the onset of motor impairment. Although not universal, they are common and may be a cause of significant distress in HD (Epping et al. 2016). Disturbed sleep is also a prominent feature of HD, substantially impairing the quality of life of both patients and their caregivers (Taylor and Bramble 1997). Currently, there is a growing awareness of the impact exerted by sleep abnormalities in HD (Bellosta Diago et al. 2017).

By using polysomnography (PSG) and actigraphy, studies have reported an increased sleep onset latency, sleep fragmentation and frequent nocturnal awakenings, reduced sleep efficiency, delayed and shortened rapid eye movement (REM) sleep, increased periodic leg movements, as well as circadian rhythm disturbances in patients with HD (Arnulf et al. 2008; Aziz et al. 2010; Emser et al. 1988; Wiegand et al. 1991; Hurelbrink, Lewis, and Barker 2005). However, it is not clear the exact nature of sleep complaints as well as their association with other symptoms of the disease. Sleep dysfunction in HD is likely to be underdiagnosed by clinicians and underreported by patients (Goodman et al. 2011). Self-report of sleep problems in HD might be reduced because patients with HD do not present excessive daytime sleepiness (Goodman et al. 2011; Aziz et al. 2010) or do not report it, mainly due to their lack of insight into their symptoms. Nevertheless, when asked directly about the quality of their sleep, up to 90% of patients acknowledge having sleep problems. The vast majority of patients (~60%) rated sleep difficulties as either "very important" or "moderately important" components of the patient's overall health problems (Taylor and Bramble 1997; Goodman, Morton, and Barker 2010).

Notwithstanding the high prevalence and the availability of clinical tools, sleep disorders are not routinely evaluated in patients with HD. The Unified Huntington Disease Rating Scale (UHDRS), which is designed to assess the functioning of HD patients, does not include questions about sleep or the circadian rhythm (Herzog-Krzywoszanska and Krzywoszanski 2019). Sleep disturbances can seriously affect daily functioning and quality of life of the patient, caregiver and family. In addition, sleep dysfunction can result in cognitive decline, mood disorders, inattentiveness and an increased risk of accidents and institutionalization. Identifying abnormalities in sleep patterns could significantly impact the management of patients.

Therefore, this chapter intends to discuss the pattern of sleep disorders in HD, as well as how sleep quality can be associated with other important clinical symptoms. We will also comment on how HD treatment is associated with sleep disruption and present the current available therapeutic options for treating sleep problems in HD.

PREVALENCE OF SLEEP PROBLEMS IN HD

Studies using self- and/or career-completion questionnaires found that 77% (Videnovic et al. 2009) to 88% (Taylor and Bramble 1997) of patients with HD report sleep problems. These problems were rated as important contributors to overall problems by 62% of them (Taylor and Bramble 1997). The most common problems were nocturnal or early morning awakening (Videnovic et al. 2009; Piano et al. 2015). The prevalence of sleep abnormalities in HD might be even higher than reported. In a PSG study, all patients with HD presented striking abnormalities in their sleep architecture, but no differences in the scores on sleep scales when compared to controls (Goodman et al. 2011). A poor correlation between subjective sleep complaints and PSG results has been described in the HD population (Piano et al. 2017).

Regarding the disease stage, sleep disturbances were found to occur at moderate-to-severe but not mild stages of HD (Hansotia, Wall, and Berendes 1985) and self-reported poor nocturnal sleep has been associated with longer disease duration (Videnovic et al. 2009). However, PSG alterations in rest-activity cycles were found in early-stage HD similar to that described in more advanced disease, which suggests that abnormalities of sleep start early in the disease course (Goodman et al. 2011). These findings were corroborated by studies showing that sleep abnormalities were present in very mild and even premanifest HD (Arnulf et al. 2008). Sleep disruption is also very common in patients with juvenile HD (JHD), being nearly ubiquitous in this population. The great majority (88%) of caretakers of patients with JHD indicated that sleep disturbances were moderate to severe and over half indicated that it was a very frequent (i.e., nightly or 'almost nightly') issue. In addition, sleep disturbance preceded HD diagnosis by several years in around half of JHD patients (Moser et al. 2017).

Data about excessive daytime sleepiness (EDS) in the HD population are inconsistent. While some studies reported no EDS (Goodman et al. 2011; Arnulf et al. 2008), others have described a prevalence as high as 50% (Videnovic et al. 2009) among HD gene carriers. When reported, daytime somnolence was associated with co-existent depression (Videnovic et al.

2009), longer disease duration and worse motor score at the UHDRS (Piano et al. 2015). Of note, self-reporting of EDS might be reduced because HD patients can lack insight about their own symptoms. Indeed, HD gene carriers demonstrated a poor correlation between subjective EDS (as assessed by the Epworth Sleepiness Scale [ESS] score) and objective daytime sleepiness (mean daytime sleep latencies at the PSG) (Arnulf et al. 2008).

SLEEP ABNORMALITIES IN HD

Virtually all patients with HD present with sleep disturbances, but there is no specific sleep pattern described for HD. The sleep characteristics are very heterogeneous and different problems can be observed in this population. The most commonly reported problems and PSG findings in HD are associated with impaired sleep maintenance, such as frequent nocturnal or early morning awakenings. In addition, insomnia and impaired sleep efficiency with increased sleep onset latency and reduced total sleep time are also frequently reported (Videnovic et al. 2009; Wiegand et al. 1991; Goodman, Morton, and Barker 2010). Patients with HD also reported increased motor nocturnal activity in comparison with control subjects (Goodman, Morton, and Barker 2010), what has been confirmed by PSG (Silvestri et al. 1995; Piano et al. 2015; Arnulf et al. 2008). They experience repeated jerking or twitching of the arms or legs during sleep, as well as fidgeting excessively in bed and wandering about at night (Goodman, Morton, and Barker 2010). Of note, periodic limb movements have been regarded as a major pathogenic mechanism of sleep disruption in HD (Piano et al. 2015).

As a result of the sleep disturbances (particularly the long sleep latency, sleep fragmentation by frequent arousal and repeated, long-lasting awakenings), the sleep structure in HD gene carriers is disturbed. The sleep pattern typically observed in adults is characterized by cycles of non-REM (NREM) sleep (60-90 min) and REM sleep (10-15 min). During a full night of sleep, these cycles repeat four to five times. The NREM phase gradually deepens from N1 to N3 stages, according to the pattern of brain electrical activity, as recorded by electroencephalography (EEG). During NREM sleep, the person is relatively still, presents high-voltage, synchronized brain waves, in addition to regular and slow breathing and heart rates, and low blood pressure. Conversely, REM sleep is physiologically similar to waking states, comprising rapid, low-voltage desynchronized brain waves and it is characterized by suppression of postural muscle tone (atonia) (Herzog-Krzywoszanska and Krzywoszanski 2019). PSG studies have shown that HD gene carriers have abnormal sleep, characterized by poorly consolidated, fragmented and irregular sleep stages with no clear stage progression of sleep cycles and extended periods of wakefulness. Moreover, multiple sleep stage shifts are commonly observed in the majority of patients. As a consequence, the periods of uninterrupted time spent in a single sleep stage are scarce (Goodman et al. 2011). Increase of light sleep and decrease of deep sleep and REM sleep have also been reported (Piano et al. 2015).

Contrary to what is observed in patients with Parkinson's disease, REM sleep behavior disorder (RBD) is not common among the HD population. Although HD patients complained about symptoms highly suggestive of a dream enactment behavior (Videnovic et al. 2009), and a few patients reported RBD symptoms, no episode of RBD was observed in a PSG study with HD gene carriers (Piano et al. 2015).

Sleep abnormalities are not associated with CAG repeat length (Arnulf et al. 2008; Hansotia, Wall, and Berendes 1985) and the etiology of the sleep disturbances in HD is not completely understood. One explanation is centered on abnormalities of the hypothalamus, thus disrupting circadian rhythms. In fact, circadian abnormalities have been consistently demonstrated in different animal models of HD, such as R6/2, R6/1, and BACHD mice, rats and drosophila transgenic models (Morton 2013). One study has shown that HD patients have disrupted night-day activity patterns that mirror the abnormalities observed in R6/2 mice. These animals displayed a circadian behavior impairment that worsened as the disease progressed, what was accompanied by a marked disruption of expression of the circadian clock genes in the suprachiasmatic nuclei (Morton et al. 2005).

Another potential mechanism underlying sleep disruption is the HD-related caudate degenerative process. An early study combining EEG, positron emission tomography (PET) and clinical findings showed that atrophy of the caudate nuclei was associated with reduced slow-wave sleep and increased time spent awake among patients with HD (Wiegand et al. 1991). Later studies have postulated that caudate degeneration observed in HD accounts for the increased arousability, increased motor activity during wake and sleep, reduction of slow-wave sleep and in particular of REM sleep and, overall, a general sleep disruption (Piano et al. 2015). The loss of specific hypothalamic neuronal populations has also been regarded as a central mechanism driving sleep disturbances, in addition to dysautonomic symptoms and weight loss (Testa and Jankovic 2019).

DIAGNOSIS OF SLEEP DISORDERS IN HD

Multiple methodologies are deployed in the diagnosis of sleep disorders in HD, including PSG, actigraphy, and self-report tools. PSG is still considered the gold standard—and the only definitive way—to diagnose sleep disorders in HD (Morton 2013) but self-report tools are a viable and cost-effective alternative. Many of the self-report tools are presented in the form of questionnaires, which are broadly applicable to other conditions such as Parkinson's Disease, Multiple System Atrophy, Progressive Supranuclear Palsy, and Restless Legs Syndrome, among others. However, sleep disorders among HD patients are still underdiagnosed, and thus the appropriate treatment is omitted. This underdiagnosis may occur due to several reasons, such as underreporting of nonmotor and sleep-related symptoms by patients and caregivers (Chaudhuri et al. 2010), or failure by clinicians to ask sufficient sleep-specific questions.

PSG, also known as a sleep study, is used alongside clinical history to diagnose sleep-related movement disorders, sleep-related breathing disorders, narcolepsy, and certain parasomnias (Kramer and Millman 2018). Components of PSG assess for sleep stages, respiratory effort, abnormal body movements, airflow, snoring, end tidal CO_2, O_2 saturation, and EKG activity. Sleep stages are measured via electroencephalography (EEG), electrooculography (EOG), and electromyography (EMG). PSG has notable limitations, including costs, extensive timeframe of study, and difficulty with accurate data collection due to uncomfortable and different sleep conditions.

Actigraphy provides a quantifiable assessment of sleep-wake cycles by measuring motor activity over a span of days to weeks. A smartwatch-like device houses an accelerometer, which monitors a patient's movement throughout the duration of the study (Kushida et al. 2005). Actigraphy provides the potential benefit of increased accuracy compared to sleep diaries and self-report tools (De Weerd 2014). It can also be measured in a home setting, which is advantageous over PSG. However, actigraphy is solely reliant on movement, a measure that only indirectly reflects measures of sleep thus posing the risk of confounding certain movements associated with awakening versus involuntary movements such as chorea. Thus, caution is necessary when interpreting data from actigraphy in HD patients (Townhill et al. 2016). Nevertheless, polysomnography data (which is not dependent on movement) has confirmed actigraphy findings in the HD population (Goodman et al. 2011).

The Pittsburgh Sleep Quality Index (PSQI) is a 19-item questionnaire designed to measure overall sleep problems during the past month. It measures variables including sleep latency, sleep duration, habitual sleep efficiency, sleep disturbances, use of sleep medication, and daytime dysfunction (Buysse et al. 1989). The PSQI also includes 5 questions for caretakers or bed partners to assess the number of times in the past month that the HD patient has experienced loud snoring, sleep apnea, leg movements, episodes of disorientation or confusion, and other episodes of restlessness during sleep. Items are scored by the survey administrator from 0 (no difficulty) to 3 (severe difficulty), and the component scores are added to create a global score ranging from 0 to 21, where a higher number indicates increased severity. A score greater than 5 signifies significant sleep disturbance with high sensitivity and specificity (Backhaus et al. 2002). While the PSQI sufficiently addresses sleep habits, it lacks coverage of other disturbances such as choreiform movements, dystonia, daytime sleepiness, akinesia, Restless Legs Syndrome, and RBD (Kurtis et al. 2018). The variables in the PSQI fit the American Academy of Sleep Medicine's diagnostic criteria of an "insomnia syndrome," defined by (1) difficulty initiating sleep or staying asleep, waking up too early, or having chronically poor quality or unrestorative sleep, (2) which occurs despite sufficient opportunity for sleep and adequate sleep circumstances, and (3) daytime impairment such as mood disturbance and fatigue due to the reported nocturnal sleep difficulty (American Academy of Sleep Medicine 2005).

The Berlin Questionnaire (BQ) is a 10-question multiple choice survey that assesses for Obstructive Sleep Apnea (OSA) (Netzer et al. 1999). It is a three-category self-report scale, which covers snoring and stoppage of breathing (category 1), EDS (category 2), and hypertension and obesity (category 3). Items are scored by category, and patients are then categorized as either low risk or high risk of having OSA. The BQ may be applied to movement disorders other than HD, such as MSA, PD, and PSP (Gama et al. 2010). It has shown modest to high sensitivity for the detection of OSA in clinical groups and in the general population, although it shows limitations due to its lack of specificity (Senaratna et al. 2017).

While the PSQI and BQ focus on nocturnal sleep disorders, HD patients also suffer from diurnal sleep disorders. Although it is not classified as a disease per se, EDS is a serious condition, which may be the result of sleep deprivation and disturbance, medication side effects, substance abuse, diseases (metabolic, neurological, or psychiatric), or central hypersomnia conditions like narcolepsy (Kurtis et al. 2018). The ESS (Johns 1991) is an 8-item questionnaire capable of measuring the risk of falling asleep during daily activities. The ESS evaluates the respondent's likelihood of falling asleep in everyday situations, such as "while watching TV" or "sitting inactive in a public place." The respondent ranks their chance of dozing on a scale from 0 to 3, with 0 indicating "no chance of dozing" and 3 indicating "high chance of dozing." A composite score of greater than 7 has diagnostic value with 75% sensitivity and 50% specificity, whereas a score greater than 10 has 52% sensitivity and 72% specificity (Johns 1994). In addition to HD, the ESS is applicable to other movement disorders such as Parkinson's Disease (Hogl et al. 2010). One limitation of the ESS is the fact that it does not include information from caregivers and outside sources (Kurtis et al. 2018).

The International Restless Legs Scale (IRLS) is a 10-question survey intended to analyze the presence and severity of a patient's RLS symptoms in the past week. RLS is defined by an uncomfortable sensation in the legs and an irresistible urge to move them, often during the evening or bedtime (NIH/NINDS 2017). It has relevance to the HD patient population due to the shared sleep disturbance symptoms and the possibility of akathisa which may be a side effect from medications used to treat chorea. The IRLS has a specific item regarding the severity of the patient's sleep disturbance due to RLS, as well as questions about the patient's tiredness, sleepiness, or mood disturbance (Walters et al. 2003). Patients answer items on a scale from 0 to 4, with 4 being the most severe response. In addition to the RLS and HD patient populations, the IRLS has been used for PSP, PD, and MSA (Gama et al. 2010).

A more modern sleep questionnaire, which was modelled after PD sleep scales, was released in 2010 in association with the University of Cambridge. This 45-item survey, unlike other widely used scales, is specific to the HD patient population. The questionnaire addresses issues including sleep duration and latency, RLS symptoms, pharmacotherapy, nocturia, and chorea, among others. It has been recommended that this scale could be used and scored in concert with the UHDRS, as the current version of UHDRS does not include questions regarding sleep symptoms (Goodman, Morton, and Barker 2010).

Self-report tools have shown utility in the diagnosis of sleep disorders in HD. However, important considerations must be made when administering questionnaires, namely the patient's ability to provide an accurate representation of perceived sleep quality. The presence or severity of the patient's cognitive status in addition to anosognosia should not be ignored when using self-report questionnaires to diagnose sleep disorders in HD.

SLEEP PROBLEMS AND CLINICAL SYMPTOMS IN HD

Sleep disturbance in HD has been associated with neurocognitive and neuropsychiatric functioning. This relationship has been examined in clinical studies and animal models of HD.

Clinical studies have primarily focused on subjective reports of sleep problems and their association with cognitive and psychiatric outcomes. Baker et al., 2016 (Baker et al. 2016) sought to investigate the association between self-reported sleep problems and cognition, psychiatric symptoms, and structural brain atrophy in premanifest and symptomatic individuals with HD using retrospective data from the IMAGE-HD project. The authors hypothesized that HD gene carriers with sleep complaints would exhibit greater cognitive dysfunction, pronounced neuropsychiatric symptoms, and increased atrophy in brain areas critical for sleep relative to HD gene carriers without reported sleep disturbance. This retrospective study analyzed data from 35 symptomatic and 35 premanifest participants. Sleep was assessed via the Beck Depression Inventory-Second Edition sleep question (BDI-II item 16), which indicates severity of change is sleep pattern in the last two weeks. The Symbol Digits Modalities Test (SDMT) and Stroop Word Reading assessed for executive functioning. Neuropsychiatric symptoms were assessed with the Hospital Anxiety and Depression Scale (HADS), Frontal Systems Behavior Scale, and Schedule of Obsessions, Compulsions, and Psychological Impulses. Volumetric analyses of the caudate, thalamus, and hypothalamus were included in the analyses. Corroborating the authors' hypothesis, HD patients with sleep complaints had worse neuropsychiatric symptoms (anxiety, depression, apathy, and disinhibition) than participants without sleep problems. In addition, participants with manifest HD who reported sleep problems also showed greater thalamic volume loss relative to manifest HD individuals without subjective sleep concerns However, no association was found between cognitive outcomes and subjective sleep problems, contradicting the study's initial assumption (Baker et al. 2016).

A more recent retrospective study also examined the association among cognitive impairment, psychiatric functioning, and patient's subjective report of sleep disturbance in early stage and pre-manifest HD patients compared to gene-negative control group (Diago et al. 2018). A strength of this study was the use of validated sleep questionnaires to assess sleep (PSQI, and the ESS). Study groups consisted of 38 mutation carries and 38 age-and-sex matched controls. Cognition and mood were assessed with the HADS, the Irritability Scale, and the cognitive section of the UHDRS. Compared to controls, HD mutation carriers had worse sleep quality, longer sleep latency, increased daytime dysfunction, and elevated levels of excessive daytime sleepiness. Poor sleep quality in HD mutation carriers was associated with cognitive dysfunction, as indicated by significantly impaired SDMT scores. Overall poor sleep quality correlated with elevated levels of depression and anxiety. Notably, the correlation between depression scores and sleep disturbances (such as pain, feeling hot, nightmares, cough, snoring) remained significant after controlling for gender, age, motor symptoms, and medications (Diago et al. 2018). These results supported previous findings showing that subjective reports of sleep disturbance in HD patients is associated with worse cognitive outcomes and increased severity of depressive and anxiety symptoms (Aziz et al. 2010; Videnovic et al. 2009; Diago et al. 2018).

To date, only a few studies have examined objective measures of sleep and cognition in the HD population. The PSG-detected sleep latency in HD patients was significantly associated with worse scores in the Luria subscale of the UHDRS, which rates executive frontal lobe dysfunction thus indicating a role of frontal lobe impairment in the delay of sleep onset in HD (Cuturic et al. 2009). A more comprehensive study conducted by Lazar et al., (2015) (Lazar et al. 2015) investigated whether sleep and metabolic disturbances were present in the premanifest disease stage and if these disturbances were associated with disease burden and early cognitive changes. Validated sleep questionnaires (Morningness-Eveningness Questionnaire, Functional Outcomes of Sleep Questionnaire, ESS, PSQI) and comprehensive sleep laboratory studies (indirect calorimetry, PSG, multiple sleep latency tests) were conducted with 30 premanifest gene carriers and 20 controls. Baseline cognitive and emotional assessment consisted of the Montreal Cognitive Assessment (MoCA), and measures of memory (Hopkins Verbal Learning Test–Revised), executive function

(Verbal Fluency Test and Trail Making Tests B), psychomotor (Trail Making Tests A and Symbol Digit Modalities Test), motor skills (Hand Tapping Test), olfactory perception (Olfactory Discrimination and Identification Test), affect (Montgomery–Asberg Depression Rating Scale, BDI-II, and Apathy Evaluation Scale). Results from a principal component analyses revealed that premanifest disease stage is characterized by sleep disturbance and no metabolic dysfunction. The observed sleep abnormalities coincided with the emergence of well-described early cognitive and affective changes. This study provided objective evidence of early sleep changes in premanifest HD gene carriers and raised the question if sleep disturbance could drive early cognitive and affective changes in the disease process (Lazar et al. 2015).

Interesting preclinical studies have also demonstrated the association between sleep disruption and cognitive impairment in HD. The transgenic R6/2 mouse model of HD exhibits disrupted circadian rhythm and cognitive decline early in the disease process that continues to worsen over time. Pallier et al., 2007 (Pallier et al. 2007), attempted to normalize sleep-wake cycles in R6/2 mice by administering daily doses of alprazolam and chloral hydrate to induce sleep and examined its effect on cognitive functioning. Results showed cognitive improvement with both modes of treatment. Alprazolam improved cognitive functioning in pre- and post-symptomatic mice in addition to regulating circadian gene expression in the suprachiasmatic nucleus, the circadian pacemaker. The authors suggested that disturbed sleep-wake cycles seen in R6/2 mice may directly contribute to the observed cognitive dysfunction (Pallier et al. 2007). In a follow-up study, Pallier & Morton (2009) (Pallier and Morton 2009) treated R6/2 mice with modafanil to improve wakefulness, which also resulted in improved cognitive function and apathy. They found that a stronger effect was achieved when both alprazolam and modafanil were used together (Pallier and Morton 2009).

HD Treatment and Sleep Disorders

So far, there is no established treatment for sleep disorders in HD. HD is a very complex disorder and the treatment of chorea and behavioral symptoms may include drugs that affect the sleep pattern.

Antidepressants are widely used to treat not only depression but also behavioral problems very common in HD such as anxiety, obsessive-compulsive behaviors, aggression, and irritability (Testa and Jankovic 2019). Antidepressants may disrupt sleep architecture mainly due to activation of serotonergic 5-HT$_2$ receptors and increased noradrenergic and dopaminergic neurotransmission. The most detrimental in this regard are serotonin and norepinephrine reuptake inhibitors (SNRI), norepinephrine reuptake inhibitors (NRI), monoamine oxidase inhibitors (MAOI), selective serotonin reuptake inhibitors (SSRI), and activating tricyclic antidepressants (TCA). On the other hand, antidepressants with antihistaminergic effects, e.g., sedating TCA, mirtazapine, mianserine, or serotonin 5-HT$_2$ receptor antagnonists, like trazodone and nefazodone rapidly improve sleep (Wichniak et al. 2017). The prevalence of insomnia and daytime somnolence is increased in patients with depression or anxiety disorders using SSRI or SNRI (especially venlafaxine) in comparison with placebo. Conversely, the prevalence of insomnia is very low in patients treated with sedating antidepressants such as mirtazapine and trazodone (Wichniak et al. 2017). However, daytime somnolence complaints are very common among these patients, which is especially worrisome in the HD population, due to the increase risk of falls.

Polysomnographic records corroborated the reported sleep changes associated with the use of antidepressants. While SSRI, SNRI, and activating TCA increase REM latency, suppress REM sleep, and impair sleep continuity, sedating antidepressants decrease sleep latency, improve sleep efficiency, increase deep sleep time, and usually have little or no effect on REM sleep. It is important to note that the use of antidepressants, including those with sedative effects, may disrupt sleep due to the induction of movement-related sleep disorders or worsening already existing conditions. For instance, SSRI, SNRI, and TCA are known to induce or aggravate sleep bruxism and impair regulation of muscle tone during REM sleep, leading to REM sleep without atonia, which may induce or worsen REM Sleep Behavior Disorder (Wichniak et al. 2017). Therefore, antidepressants (especially venlafaxine) should not be used in patients suffering from RBD because they can aggravate the symptoms (Herzog-Krzywoszanska and Krzywoszanski 2019). Moreover, antidepressants such as mianserin, mirtazapine, SSRI and venlafaxine are associated with treatment-emergent restless legs syndrome (Wichniak et al. 2017). It is worth mentioning the effects of antidepressants on sleep were described for patients with depression and/or anxiety disorders and different outcomes might occur in the HD population.

Sleep disturbances are among the main side effects associated with the use of the VMAT2 inhibitor tetrabenazine, the first FDA-approved medication for the treatment of chorea secondary to HD. A significant increase in reports of sedation/somnolence and insomnia were reported by patients using tetrabenzine in comparison with placebo (Frank 2009; Yero and Rey 2008). Somnolence was the most commonly reported adverse event associated with the use deutetrabenazine, an isotopic isomer of tetrabenazine with improved pharmacokinetic profile (Huntington Study et al. 2016).

Although tetrabenazine and deutetetrabenazine are the only two FDA approved medications approved for the control of chorea in HD (Mestre et al. 2009), antipsychotics are the most commonly prescribed drugs for treating chorea in addition to alleviating severe aggressive behaviors in HD (Mason and Barker 2016). The wide use of antipsychotics can be explained at least in part because of the important cost differences between VMAT2 inhibitors and antipsychotics (Testa and Jankovic 2019). The most common used antipsychotics are olanzapine, sulpiride, amisulpiride haloperidol, and risperidone and they are all associated with sedation (Mason and Barker 2016). Dopaminergic drugs are also commonly use to treat Parkinsonism in HD. All dopaminergic drugs, including levodopa, are associated with sedative effects, which can be mitigated by dose adjustment or changing the drugs prescribed to patients (Herzog-Krzywoszanska and Krzywoszanski 2019). Of note, when administered at bedtime, the medications used to reduce chorea that present with sedative properties can improve insomnia secondary to the attenuation of chorea and anxiety or agitation from movements in HD (Testa and Jankovic 2019).

Benzodiazepines are also commonly used to treat anxiety and insomnia, in addition to motor disturbances in HD (Mason and Barker 2016), but the potential for abuse and the severe adverse effects dampens enthusiasm for the use of such drugs. Benzodiazepines may negatively impact balance and they have an enormous cognitive impact; therefore they should be started at a very low dose, titrated up gradually, and tapered off when no longer necessary (Testa and Jankovic 2019).

Unfortunately, there is no systematic study of sleep disorders treatment in HD (Morton 2013). Melatonin - a neurohormone that has been shown to improve sleep disturbances in the elderly as well as in Parkinson's disease - might be beneficial. Here again, the efficacy is not well established, but the use of melatonin is unlikely to result in deleterious side effects in HD patients (Morton 2013). The use of melatonin in supported by findings that patients with HD present abnormal pattern of melatonin release / decreased melatonin levels (Adamczak-Ratajczak et al. 2017; Kalliolia et al. 2014). In addition to modulating the circadian rhythmicity, melatonin might be neuroprotective due to its potent scavenger properties of oxygen and nitrogen reactive species, anti-inflammatory and immune-enhancing activities (Sanchez-Barcelo et al. 2017).

Non-pharmacological therapies can be very effective, especially for nonmanifest individuals. These include general health measures such as exercise, appropriate diet, stress management, and social engagement (Testa and Jankovic 2019). Patients should be encouraged to establish sleep hygiene measures, such as minimize caffeine intake, avoid or abolish nicotine and alcohol use, avoid napping during the daytime, and adopt a regular schedule for sleeping and waking up (Morton 2013). Cognitive Behavior Therapy (CBT), usually a combination of multi-modality interventions is a standard of therapeutic care in patients with chronic insomnia. Although its efficacy has not been tested specifically in patients with HD, given the prevalence of psychiatric symptoms in this population, it may be considered as a viable alternative (Morgenthaler et al. 2006).

Recently, expert-based recommendations were published as an attempt to provide guidelines for the treatment of neuropsychiatric symptoms and sleep problems in HD. The experts agreed that the choice of drug for treating sleep impairment in HD is often dependent on presence of coexisting disease symptoms and may vary with stage of disease. In addition, they noted that drugs used in the treatment of sleep disorders in HD may be associated with adverse effects that mimic symptoms of HD (Anderson et al. 2018). The expert-based recommendations are summarized below:

- General recommendations: Treat co-morbid conditions, especially psychiatric symptoms, or substance use that can contribute to sleep disruption. Adjust dosing schedule of drugs that may contribute either to daytime sleepiness or nocturnal insomnia.
- Behavioral Treatment Recommendations: Encourage the implementation of good sleep hygiene as the initial step for treating sleep disturbances.
- Pharmacologic Treatment Recommendations: Melatonin is a pharmacologic option particularly when there is evidence of circadian rhythm disorder. Sedating antidepressants (e.g.,: mirtazapine or trazodone) or sedating antipsychotics (e.g.,: olanzapine and quetiapine) are pharmacologic options for treating insomnia in HD. Clomipramine is a pharmacologic option if this drug is needed for management of coexisting obsessive perseverative symptoms. The use of benzodiazepines is discouraged unless all other options have failed (Anderson et al. 2018).

CONCLUSION

In reviewing the current available studies, we can conclude that sleep problems are almost universal among the HD population. There is no specific pattern of sleep described in individuals with HD, however, patients usually report impaired sleep maintenance, frequent awakenings, insomnia and decreased sleep efficiency. PSG data confirm the patients' complaints, showing that HD gene carriers have disturbed sleep, characterized by poorly consolidated, fragmented and irregular sleep stages with no clear stage progression of sleep cycles and extended periods of wakefulness. Given the high prevalence and the impact of sleep problems on cognitive and psychiatric symptoms, the diagnosis and treatment of disrupted sleep is paramount when caring for individuals with HD. Identification and treatment of psychiatric symptoms and other nonmotor problems is recommended. In addition, patients should be encouraged to follow good sleep hygiene practices. Appropriate sleep hygiene including appropriate bedding and environmental modifications should also be implemented (Testa and Jankovic 2019). If pharmacologic intervention is needed, melatonin is recommended before any other prescription because of the reduced side effect burden and no potential dependency, unlike other sleep medications. The depressed patients with clinically significant insomnia should be treated with a sedating antidepressant, reducing the need to use benzodiazepines or sedative hypnotics. When treating HD related sleep dysfunction special attention should be paid to addressing HD motor symptoms as well. Treating excessive involuntary movements or Parkinsonism can prevent or diminish falls out of bed or while ambulating to the restroom at night. Finally, reviewing the medication list is imperative to reduce the use of medications that might impair sleep quality or quantity. HD is a complex neurodegenerative disease that affects multiple systems, addressing sleep quality and quantity with pharmacologic and nonpharmacologic treatments can positively impact quality of life.

REFERENCES

Adamczak-Ratajczak, A., J. Kupsz, M. Owecki, D. Zielonka, A. Sowinska, Z. Checinska-Maciejewska, H. Krauss, S. Michalak, and M. Gibas-Dorna. 2017. "Circadian rhythms of melatonin and cortisol in manifest Huntington's disease and in acute cortical ischemic stroke." *J Physiol Pharmacol* 68 (4): 539-546. http://www.ncbi.nlm.nih.gov/pubmed/29151070.

AmericanAcademyofSleepMedicine. 2005. *"International Classification of Sleep Disorders: Diagnostic and Coding Manual."* Westchester, IL: American Academy of Sleep Medicine.

Anderson, K. E., E. van Duijn, D. Craufurd, C. Drazinic, M. Edmondson, N. Goodman, D. van Kammen, C. Loy, J. Priller, and L. V. Goodman. 2018. "Clinical Management of Neuropsychiatric Symptoms of Huntington Disease: Expert-Based Consensus Guidelines on Agitation, Anxiety, Apathy, Psychosis and Sleep Disorders." *J Huntingtons Dis* 7 (3): 355-366. https://doi.org/10.3233/JHD-180293. https://www.ncbi. nlm.nih.gov/pubmed/30040737.

Arnulf, I., J. Nielsen, E. Lohmann, J. Schiefer, E. Wild, P. Jennum, E. Konofal, M. Walker, D. Oudiette, S. Tabrizi, and A. Durr. 2008. "Rapid eye movement sleep disturbances in Huntington disease." *Arch Neurol* 65 (4): 482-8. https://doi.org/10.1001/archneur.65.4.482. http://www. ncbi.nlm.nih.gov/pubmed/18413470.

Aziz, N. A., G. V. Anguelova, J. Marinus, G. J. Lammers, and R. A. Roos. 2010. "Sleep and circadian rhythm alterations correlate with depression and cognitive impairment in Huntington's disease." *Parkinsonism Relat Disord* 16 (5): 345-50. https://doi.org/10.1016/j.parkreldis.2010.02.009. http://www.ncbi.nlm.nih.gov/pubmed/20236854.

Backhaus, J., K. Junghanns, A. Broocks, D. Riemann, and F. Hohagen. 2002. "Test-retest reliability and validity of the Pittsburgh Sleep Quality Index in primary insomnia." *J Psychosom Res* 53 (3): 737-40. https://www.ncbi.nlm.nih.gov/pubmed/12217446.

Baker, C. R., D. Jf Dominguez, J. C. Stout, S. Gabery, A. Churchyard, P. Chua, G. F. Egan, A. Petersen, N. Georgiou-Karistianis, and G. R. Poudel. 2016. "Subjective sleep problems in Huntington's disease: A pilot investigation of the relationship to brain structure, neurocognitive, and neuropsychiatric function." *J Neurol Sci* 364: 148-53. https://doi.org/10.1016/j.jns.2016.03.021. https://www.ncbi. nlm. nih.gov/pubmed/27084236.

Bellosta Diago, E., J. Perez Perez, S. Santos Lasaosa, A. Viloria Alebesque, S. Martinez Horta, J. Kulisevsky, and J. Lopez Del Val. 2017. "Circadian rhythm and autonomic dysfunction in presymptomatic and early Huntington's disease." *Parkinsonism Relat Disord* 44: 95-100. https://doi.org/10.1016/j.parkreldis.2017.09.013. http://www.ncbi.nlm.nih.gov/pubmed/28935191.

Buysse, D. J., C. F. Reynolds, 3rd, T. H. Monk, S. R. Berman, and D. J. Kupfer. 1989. "The Pittsburgh Sleep Quality Index: a new instrument for psychiatric practice and research." *Psychiatry Res* 28 (2): 193-213. http://www.ncbi.nlm.nih.gov/pubmed/2748771.

Chaudhuri, K. R., C. Prieto-Jurcynska, Y. Naidu, T. Mitra, B. Frades-Payo, S. Tluk, A. Ruessmann, P. Odin, G. Macphee, F. Stocchi, W. Ondo, K. Sethi, A. H. Schapira, J. C. Martinez Castrillo, and P. Martinez-Martin. 2010. "The nondeclaration of nonmotor symptoms of Parkinson's disease to health care professionals: an international study using the nonmotor symptoms questionnaire." *Mov Disord* 25 (6): 704-9. https://doi.org/10.1002/mds.22868. https://www.ncbi.nlm.nih.gov/pubmed/20437539.

Cuturic, M., R. K. Abramson, D. Vallini, E. M. Frank, and M. Shamsnia. 2009. "Sleep patterns in patients with Huntington's disease and their unaffected first-degree relatives: a brief report." *Behav Sleep Med* 7 (4): 245-54. https://doi.org/10.1080/15402000903190215. https://www.ncbi.nlm.nih.gov/pubmed/19787493.

De Weerd, A. W. 2014. "Actigraphy, the alternative way?" *Front Psychiatry* 5: 155. https://doi.org/10.3389/fpsyt.2014.00155. https://www.ncbi.nlm.nih.gov/pubmed/25520671.

Diago, E. B., S. Martinez-Horta, S. S. Lasaosa, A. V. Alebesque, J. Perez-Perez, J. Kulisevsky, and J. L. Del Val. 2018. "Circadian Rhythm, Cognition, and Mood Disorders in Huntington's Disease." *J Huntingtons Dis* 7 (2): 193-198. https://doi.org/10.3233/JHD-180291. https://www.ncbi.nlm.nih.gov/pubmed/29843249.

Duff, K., J. S. Paulsen, L. J. Beglinger, D. R. Langbehn, C. Wang, J. C. Stout, C. A. Ross, E. Aylward, N. E. Carlozzi, S. Queller, and H. D. Investigators of the Huntington Study Group Predict. 2010. ""Frontal" behaviors before the diagnosis of Huntington's disease and their relationship to markers of disease progression: evidence of early lack of awareness." *J Neuropsychiatry Clin Neurosci* 22 (2): 196-207.

https://doi.org/10.1176/appi.neuropsych.22.2.196.   10.1176/jnp.2010.
22.2.196. http://www.ncbi.nlm.nih.gov/pubmed/20463114.

Emser, W., M. Brenner, T. Stober, and K. Schimrigk. 1988. "Changes in
nocturnal sleep in Huntington's and Parkinson's disease." *J Neurol* 235
(3): 177-9. http://www.ncbi.nlm.nih.gov/pubmed/2966851.

Epping, E. A., J. I. Kim, D. Craufurd, T. M. Brashers-Krug, K. E. Anderson,
E. McCusker, J. Luther, J. D. Long, J. S. Paulsen, Predict-Hd
Investigators, and Group Coordinators of the Huntington Study. 2016.
"Longitudinal Psychiatric Symptoms in Prodromal Huntington's
Disease: A Decade of Data." *Am J Psychiatry* 173 (2): 184-92.
https://doi.org/10.1176/appi.ajp.2015.14121551. http://www.ncbi.nlm.
nih.gov/pubmed/26472629.

Frank, S. 2009. "Tetrabenazine as anti-chorea therapy in Huntington
disease: an open-label continuation study. Huntington Study
Group/TETRA-HD Investigators." *BMC Neurol* 9: 62. https://doi.
org/10.1186/1471-2377-9-62. https://www.ncbi.nlm.nih.gov/pubmed/
20021666.

Gama, R. L., D. G. Tavora, R. C. Bomfim, C. E. Silva, V. M. de Bruin, and
P. F. de Bruin. 2010. "Sleep disturbances and brain MRI morphometry
in Parkinson's disease, multiple system atrophy and progressive
supranuclear palsy - a comparative study." *Parkinsonism Relat Disord*
16 (4): 275-9. https://doi.org/10.1016/j.parkreldis.2010.01.002.
https://www.ncbi.nlm.nih.gov/pubmed/20185356.

Goodman, A. O., A. J. Morton, and R. A. Barker. 2010. "Identifying sleep
disturbances in Huntington's disease using a simple disease-focused
questionnaire." *PLoS Curr* 2: RRN1189. https://doi.org/10.1371/
currents.RRN1189. http://www.ncbi.nlm.nih.gov/pubmed/20972477.

Goodman, A. O., L. Rogers, S. Pilsworth, C. J. McAllister, J. M. Shneerson,
A. J. Morton, and R. A. Barker. 2011. "Asymptomatic sleep
abnormalities are a common early feature in patients with Huntington's
disease." *Curr Neurol Neurosci Rep* 11 (2): 211-7. https:/
doi.org/10.1007/s11910-010-0163-x. http://www.ncbi.nlm.nih.gov/
pubmed/21103960.

Hansotia, P., R. Wall, and J. Berendes. 1985. "Sleep disturbances and severity of Huntington's disease." *Neurology* 35 (11): 1672-4. https://doi.org/10.1212/wnl.35.11.1672. https://www.ncbi.nlm.nih.gov/pubmed/2932657.

Herzog-Krzywoszanska, R., and L. Krzywoszanski. 2019. "Sleep Disorders in Huntington's Disease." *Front Psychiatry* 10: 221. https://doi.org/10.3389/fpsyt.2019.00221. https://www.ncbi.nlm.nih.gov/pubmed/31031659.

Hogl, B., I. Arnulf, C. Comella, J. Ferreira, A. Iranzo, B. Tilley, C. Trenkwalder, W. Poewe, O. Rascol, C. Sampaio, G. T. Stebbins, A. Schrag, and C. G. Goetz. 2010. "Scales to assess sleep impairment in Parkinson's disease: critique and recommendations." *Mov Disord* 25 (16): 2704-16. https://doi.org/10.1002/mds.23190. https://www.ncbi.nlm.nih.gov/pubmed/20931631.

Huntington Study, Group, S. Frank, C. M. Testa, D. Stamler, E. Kayson, C. Davis, M. C. Edmondson, S. Kinel, B. Leavitt, D. Oakes, C. O'Neill, C. Vaughan, J. Goldstein, M. Herzog, V. Snively, J. Whaley, C. Wong, G. Suter, J. Jankovic, J. Jimenez-Shahed, C. Hunter, D. O. Claassen, O. C. Roman, V. Sung, J. Smith, S. Janicki, R. Clouse, M. Saint-Hilaire, A. Hohler, D. Turpin, R. C. James, R. Rodriguez, K. Rizer, K. E. Anderson, H. Heller, A. Carlson, S. Criswell, B. A. Racette, F. J. Revilla, F. Nucifora, Jr., R. L. Margolis, M. Ong, T. Mendis, N. Mendis, C. Singer, M. Quesada, J. S. Paulsen, T. Brashers-Krug, A. Miller, J. Kerr, R. M. Dubinsky, C. Gray, S. A. Factor, E. Sperin, E. Molho, M. Eglow, S. Evans, R. Kumar, C. Reeves, A. Samii, S. Chouinard, M. Beland, B. L. Scott, P. T. Hickey, S. Esmail, W. L. Fung, C. Gibbons, L. Qi, A. Colcher, C. Hackmyer, A. McGarry, K. Klos, M. Gudesblatt, L. Fafard, L. Graffitti, D. P. Schneider, R. Dhall, J. M. Wojcieszek, K. LaFaver, A. Duker, E. Neefus, H. Wilson-Perez, D. Shprecher, P. Wall, K. A. Blindauer, L. Wheeler, J. T. Boyd, E. Houston, E. S. Farbman, P. Agarwal, S. W. Eberly, A. Watts, P. N. Tariot, A. Feigin, S. Evans, C. Beck, C. Orme, J. Edicola, and E. Christopher. 2016. "Effect of Deutetrabenazine on Choreaamongg Patients with Huntington Disease: A Randomized Clinical Trial." *JAMA* 316 (1): 40-50.

https://doi.org/10.1001/jama.2016.8655. http://www.ncbi.nlm.nih.gov/pubmed/27380342.

Hurelbrink, C. B., S. J. Lewis, and R. A. Barker. 2005. "The use of the Actiwatch-Neurologica system to objectively assess the involuntary movements and sleep-wake activity in patients with mild-moderate Huntington's disease." *J Neurol* 252 (6): 642-7. https://doi.org/10.1007/s00415-005-0709-z. https://www.ncbi.nlm.nih.gov/pubmed/15742112.

Johns, M. W. 1991. "A new method for measuring daytime sleepiness: the Epworth sleepiness scale." *Sleep* 14 (6): 540-5.

Johns, M. W. 1994. "Sleepiness in different situations measured by the Epworth Sleepiness Scale." *Sleep* 17 (8): 703-10. https://doi.org/10.1093/sleep/17.8.703. https://www.ncbi.nlm.nih.gov/pubmed/7701181.

Kalliolia, E., E. Silajdzic, R. Nambron, N. R. Hill, A. Doshi, C. Frost, H. Watt, P. Hindmarsh, M. Bjorkqvist, and T. T. Warner. 2014. "Plasma melatonin is reduced in Huntington's disease." *Mov Disord* 29 (12): 1511-5. https://doi.org/10.1002/mds.26003. http://www.ncbi.nlm.nih.gov/pubmed/25164424.

Kramer, N. R., and R. P. Millman. 2018. "*Overview of polysomnography in adults.*" Wolters Kluwer. Accessed 07/15/2019. https://www.uptodate.com/contents/search.

Kurtis, M. M., R. Balestrino, C. Rodriguez-Blazquez, M. J. Forjaz, and P. Martinez-Martin. 2018. "A Review of Scales to Evaluate Sleep Disturbances in Movement Disorders." *Front Neurol* 9: 369. https://doi.org/10.3389/fneur.2018.00369. https://www.ncbi.nlm.nih.gov/pubmed/29896152.

Kushida, C. A., M. R. Littner, T. Morgenthaler, C. A. Alessi, D. Bailey, J. Coleman, Jr., L. Friedman, M. Hirshkowitz, S. Kapen, M. Kramer, T. Lee-Chiong, D. L. Loube, J. Owens, J. P. Pancer, and M. Wise. 2005. "Practice parameters for the indications for polysomnography and related procedures: an update for 2005." *Sleep* 28 (4): 499-521. http://www.ncbi.nlm.nih.gov/pubmed/16171294.

Lazar, A. S., F. Panin, A. O. Goodman, S. E. Lazic, Z. I. Lazar, S. L. Mason, L. Rogers, P. R. Murgatroyd, L. P. Watson, P. Singh, B. Borowsky, J. M. Shneerson, and R. A. Barker. 2015. "Sleep deficits but no metabolic deficits in premanifest Huntington's disease." *Ann Neurol* 78 (4): 630-48. https://doi.org/10.1002/ana.24495. https://www.ncbi.nlm.nih.gov/pubmed/26224419.

Mason, S. L., and R. A. Barker. 2016. "Advancing pharmacotherapy for treating Huntington's disease: a review of the existing literature." *Expert Opin Pharmacother* 17 (1): 41-52. https://doi.org/10.1517/1465 6566.2016.1109630. https://www.ncbi.nlm.nih.gov/pubmed/2653 6068.

Mestre, T., J. Ferreira, M. M. Coelho, M. Rosa, and C. Sampaio. 2009. "Therapeutic interventions for symptomatic treatment in Huntington's disease." *Cochrane Database Syst Rev* (3): CD006456. https://doi.org/10.1002/14651858.CD006456.pub2. https://www.ncbi.nlm.nih.gov/pubmed/19588393.

Morgenthaler, T., M. Kramer, C. Alessi, L. Friedman, B. Boehlecke, T. Brown, J. Coleman, V. Kapur, T. Lee-Chiong, J. Owens, J. Pancer, T. Swick, and Medicine American Academy of Sleep. 2006. "Practice parameters for the psychological and behavioral treatment of insomnia: an update. An american academy of sleep medicine report." *Sleep* 29 (11): 1415-9. https://www.ncbi.nlm.nih.gov/pubmed/17162987.

Morton, A. J. 2013. "Circadian and sleep disorder in Huntington's disease." *Exp Neurol* 243: 34-44. https://doi.org/10.1016/j.expneurol.2012.10.014. http://www.ncbi.nlm.nih.gov/pubmed/23099415.

Morton, A. J., N. I. Wood, M. H. Hastings, C. Hurelbrink, R. A. Barker, and E. S. Maywood. 2005. "Disintegration of the sleep-wake cycle and circadian timing in Huntington's disease." *J Neurosci* 25 (1): 157-63. https://doi.org/10.1523/JNEUROSCI.3842-04.2005. https://www.ncbi.nlm.nih.gov/pubmed/15634777.

Moser, A. D., E. Epping, P. Espe-Pfeifer, E. Martin, L. Zhorne, K. Mathews, M. Nance, D. Hudgell, O. Quarrell, and P. Nopoulos. 2017. "A survey-based study identifies common but unrecognized symptoms in a large series of juvenile Huntington's disease." *Neurodegener Dis Manag* 7

(5): 307-315. https://doi.org/10.2217/nmt-2017-0019. http://www.ncbi.nlm.nih.gov/pubmed/29043929.

Netzer, N. C., R. A. Stoohs, C. M. Netzer, K. Clark, and K. P. Strohl. 1999. "Using the Berlin Questionnaire to identify patients at risk for the sleep apnea syndrome." *Ann Intern Med* 131 (7): 485-91. https://doi.org/10.7326/0003-4819-131-7-199910050-00002. https://www.ncbi.nlm.nih.gov/pubmed/10507956.

NIH/NINDS. 2017. "Restless Legs Syndrome Fact Sheet." *NIH/NINDS*. Accessed 07/15/2019. https://www.ninds.nih.gov/disorders/patient-caregiver-education/fact-sheets/restless-legs-syndrome-fact-sheet.

Pallier, P. N., E. S. Maywood, Z. Zheng, J. E. Chesham, A. N. Inyushkin, R. Dyball, M. H. Hastings, and A. J. Morton. 2007. "Pharmacological imposition of sleep slows cognitive decline and reverses dysregulation of circadian gene expression in a transgenic mouse model of Huntington's disease." *J Neurosci* 27 (29): 7869-78. https://doi.org/10.1523/JNEUROSCI.0649-07.2007. https://www.ncbi.nlm.nih.gov/pubmed/17634381.

Pallier, P. N., and A. J. Morton. 2009. "Management of sleep/wake cycles improves cognitive function in a transgenic mouse model of Huntington's disease." *Brain Res* 1279: 90-8. https://doi.org/10.1016/j.brainres.2009.03.072. https://www.ncbi.nlm.nih.gov/pubmed/ 19450569.

Piano, C., G. Della Marca, A. Losurdo, C. Imperatori, M. Solito, G. Calandra-Buonaura, F. Provini, P. Cortelli, and A. R. Bentivoglio. 2017. "Subjective Assessment of Sleep in Huntington Disease: Reliability of Sleep Questionnaires Compared to Polysomnography." *Neurodegener Dis* 17 (6): 330-337. https://doi.org/10.1159/000480701. https://www.ncbi.nlm.nih.gov/pubmed/29169178.

Piano, C., A. Losurdo, G. Della Marca, M. Solito, G. Calandra-Buonaura, F. Provini, A. R. Bentivoglio, and P. Cortelli. 2015. "Polysomnographic Findings and Clinical Correlates in Huntington Disease: A Cross-Sectional Cohort Study." *Sleep* 38 (9): 1489-95. https://doi.org/10.5665/sleep.4996. https://www.ncbi.nlm.nih.gov/pubmed/25845698.

Reiner, A., I. Dragatsis, and P. Dietrich. 2011. "Genetics and neuropathology of Huntington's disease." *Int Rev Neurobiol* 98: 325-72. https://doi.org/10.1016/B978-0-12-381328-2.00014-6. http://www. ncbi.nlm.nih.gov/pubmed/21907094.

Ross, C. A., E. H. Aylward, E. J. Wild, D. R. Langbehn, J. D. Long, J. H. Warner, R. I. Scahill, B. R. Leavitt, J. C. Stout, J. S. Paulsen, R. Reilmann, P. G. Unschuld, A. Wexler, R. L. Margolis, and S. J. Tabrizi. 2014. "Huntington disease: natural history, biomarkers and prospects for therapeutics." *Nat Rev Neurol* 10 (4): 204-16. https://doi.org/ 10.1038/nrneurol.2014.24. http://www.ncbi.nlm.nih.gov/pubmed/ 24614516.

Ross, C. A., and S. J. Tabrizi. 2011. "Huntington's disease: from molecular pathogenesis to clinical treatment." *Lancet Neurol* 10 (1): 83-98. https://doi.org/10.1016/S1474-4422(10)70245-3. http://www.ncbi.nlm. nih.gov/pubmed/21163446.

Sanchez-Barcelo, E. J., N. Rueda, M. D. Mediavilla, C. Martinez-Cue, and R. J. Reiter. 2017. "Clinical Uses of Melatonin in Neurological Diseases and Mental and Behavioural Disorders." *Curr Med Chem* 24 (35): 3851-3878. https://doi.org/10.2174/0929867324666170718105557. https://www.ncbi.nlm.nih.gov/pubmed/28721826.

Senaratna, C. V., J. L. Perret, M. C. Matheson, C. J. Lodge, A. J. Lowe, R. Cassim, M. A. Russell, J. A. Burgess, G. S. Hamilton, and S. C. Dharmage. 2017. "Validity of the Berlin questionnaire in detecting obstructive sleep apnea: A systematic review and meta-analysis." *Sleep Med Rev* 36: 116-124. https://doi.org/10.1016/j.smrv.2017.04.001. https://www.ncbi.nlm.nih.gov/pubmed/28599983.

Silvestri, R., M. Raffaele, P. De Domenico, A. Tisano, G. Mento, C. Casella, M. C. Tripoli, S. Serra, and R. Di Perri. 1995. "Sleep features in Tourette's syndrome, neuroacanthocytosis and Huntington's chorea." *Neurophysiol Clin* 25 (2): 66-77. https://doi.org/10.1016/ 0987-7053(96)81034-3. https://www.ncbi.nlm.nih.gov/pubmed/7603 414.

Taylor, N., and D. Bramble. 1997. "Sleep disturbance and Huntingdon's disease." *Br J Psychiatry* 171: 393. http://www.ncbi.nlm.nih.gov/pubmed/9373439.

Testa, C. M., and J. Jankovic. 2019. "Huntington disease: A quarter century of progress since the gene discovery." *J Neurol Sci* 396: 52-68. https://doi.org/10.1016/j.jns.2018.09.022.   https://www.ncbi.nlm.nih.gov/pubmed/30419368.

Townhill, J., A. C. Hughes, B. Thomas, M. E. Busse, K. Price, S. B. Dunnett, M. H. Hastings, and A. E. Rosser. 2016. "Using Actiwatch to monitor circadian rhythm disturbance in Huntington' disease: A cautionary note." *J Neurosci Methods* 265: 13-8. https://doi.org/10.1016/j.jneumeth.2016.01.009.   https://www.ncbi.nlm.nih.gov/pubmed/2677 4754.

Videnovic, A., S. Leurgans, W. Fan, J. Jaglin, and K. M. Shannon. 2009. "Daytime somnolence and nocturnal sleep disturbances in Huntington disease." *Parkinsonism Relat Disord* 15 (6): 471-4. https://doi.org/10.1016/j.parkreldis.2008.10.002.   https://www.ncbi.nlm.nih.gov/pubmed/19041273.

Walters, A. S., C. LeBrocq, A. Dhar, W. Hening, R. Rosen, R. P. Allen, C. Trenkwalder, and Group International Restless Legs Syndrome Study. 2003. "Validation of the International Restless Legs Syndrome Study Group rating scale for restless legs syndrome." *Sleep Med* 4 (2): 121-32. https://www.ncbi.nlm.nih.gov/pubmed/14592342.

Wichniak, A., A. Wierzbicka, M. Walecka, and W. Jernajczyk. 2017. "Effects of Antidepressants on Sleep." *Curr Psychiatry Rep* 19 (9): 63. https://doi.org/10.1007/s11920-017-0816-4. https://www.ncbi.nlm.nih.gov/pubmed/28791566.

Wiegand, M., A. A. Moller, C. J. Lauer, S. Stolz, W. Schreiber, M. Dose, and J. C. Krieg. 1991. "Nocturnal sleep in Huntington's disease." *J Neurol* 238 (4): 203-8. http://www.ncbi.nlm.nih.gov/pubmed/1832711.

Yero, T., and J. A. Rey. 2008. "Tetrabenazine (Xenazine), An FDA-Approved Treatment Option For Huntington's Disease-Related Chorea." *P T* 33 (12): 690-4. https://www.ncbi.nlm.nih.gov/pubmed/19750050.

In: Living with Huntington's Disease   ISBN: 978-1-53616-729-0
Editor: Sherman Howell   © 2020 Nova Science Publishers, Inc.

Chapter 2

CLINICAL TRIALS IN HD: LESSONS LEARNED, PROGRESS, AND PERSPECTIVES

Natalia P. Rocha[1,2], Gabriela D. Colpo[3], Dylan May[4], Antonio L. Teixeira[3] and Erin Furr Stimming[2,5]

[1]Mitchell Center for Alzheimer's disease and Related Brain Disorders, Department of Neurology, The University of Texas Health Science Center, Houston, TX, US

[2]HDSA Center of Excellence at University of Texas Health Science Center at Houston, Houston, TX, US

[3]Neuropsychiatry Program, Department of Psychiatry and Behavioral Sciences, The University of Texas Health Science Center at Houston, Houston, TX, US

[4]University of Virginia

[5]Department of Neurology, The University of Texas Health Science Center, Houston, TX, US

ABSTRACT

Although HD is categorized as a movement disorder, the wide range of non-motor symptoms including cognitive impairment and behavioral abnormalities are considered by patients and their caregivers to be just as disabling as the motor symptoms. Motor and nonmotor symptomatic treatment is an important consideration to improve both functionality and quality of life in HD. A variety of symptomatic treatments are currently available. Pharmacological options for the motor symptoms include tetrabenazine and deutetrabenazine – the only two FDA-approved drugs for HD related chorea, neuroleptics, gabaergic and antiglutaminergic medications are often used off label. Antidepressants and neuroleptics are also used to treat the neuropsychiatiric symptoms. Interdisciplinary, non-pharmacological options are available such as, psychotherapy, physical, occupational and speech therapy, genetic counseling, social work and nutritional services. However, there is currently no approved disease-modifying therapy for HD. After the discovery of the genetic cause for HD 26 years ago, great efforts have been made to identify a treatment capable of modifying the disease course. Recent advances in therapeutic strategies promise an exciting era for clinical trials in HD. Increased recognition of the phenotypic variability in HD can also improve the symptomatic treatment goals. This endeavor will be coupled with advances in novel therapeutics, including strategies in lowering the mutant huntingtin protein and targeting the *HTT* gene. Future novel HD treatments are focused on positively impacting both quality of life and longevity in individuals with HD, in addition to contributing to research in other neurodegenerative disorders. This chapter will present the past, current and future clinical trials targeting both symptomatic and disease-modifying treatments for HD.

INTRODUCTION

Huntington's disease (HD) is a neurodegenerative disease classically characterized by a triad of signs and symptoms: 1) a complex movement disorder consisting of involuntary movements (mainly chorea), and impairment of voluntary movements (including incoordination, slowing of saccades, bradykinesia, and rigidity); 2) a cognitive disorder, predominantly characterized by a dysexecutive syndrome and cognitive deficits at the intersection between cognitive and psychiatric realms of function; 3) a variety of behavioral problems including apathy, irritability, depression, and anxiety (C.A. Ross, Aylward, et al. 2014; T.A. Mestre 2019).

The causative mutation was identified 26 years ago – HD is a highly penetrant, autosomal dominant genetic disease caused by a CAG trinucleotide repeat expansion in the huntingtin (*HTT*) gene (located on the short arm of chromosome 4 (4p16.3)] (The Huntington's Disease Collaborative Research Group 1993). The CAG repeat expansion in the *HTT* gene exon 1 is translated into an expanded polyglutamine repeat in the huntingtin protein (HTT), resulting in a mutant HTT (mHTT) (Testa and Jankovic 2019). Although there is no cure for this devastating disorder, the discovery of the gene that causes HD has been a major milestone in HD research, and multiple disease-modifying studies have subsequently been conducted. In parallel with trials aimed at changing the disease course, advances have also been made in HD symptomatic treatment. While HD-specific treatment recommendations are limited, the relative wealth of available symptomatic interventions makes this a key area of opportunity for clinical care (Testa and Jankovic 2019). Increased recognition of the phenotypic variability in HD can also improve the symptomatic treatment goals. This chapter will present the past, current and future clinical trials registered at clinicaltrials.gov. Table 1 summarizes that past clinical trials and Table 2 the current/future trials targeting both disease-modifying and symptomatic therapies in HD.

DISEASE-MODIFYING THERAPIES IN HUNTINGTON'S DISEASE

Despite multiple attempts to identify an effective disease-modifying therapy for HD, an approved disease modifying therapy remains elusive. Various compounds have been studied, including novel approaches such as immune therapies targeting the immune dysregulation in HD and interventions with multiple targets. More recently, due to the rapid advances in gene modifying technology, novel promising strategies have been proposed, such as reducing the amount of mHTT, inhibition of synthesis of mHTT, and modulation of HTT homeostasis.

mHTT Lowering Therapies

Lowering mHTT levels has become one of the most promising therapeutic options aimed at disease modification. These strategies focused on inhibiting mRNA synthesis by blocking transcription (Zinc finger motif proteins), avoiding post-transcriptional processes and stimulating early mRNA degradation (antisense oligonucleotides, ASO) or inhibiting mRNA translation (small interfering RNA, siRNA) (T.A. Mestre 2019).

After positive results in preclinical studies (Stanek et al. 2013), the first human clinical trial with ASO therapy targeted at lowering HTT was performed by Ionis Pharmaceuticals in collaboration with Roche (NCT02519036). The clinical trial evaluated the safety, tolerability, pharmacokinetics, and pharmacodynamics of multiple ascending doses of IONIS-HTTRx lumbar intrathecal administration at 4-week intervals over a 13-week treatment period in 46 patients with early manifest HD. IONIS-HTTRx* is a non-allele specific human HTT ASO and thus targets both wild type HTT (wtHTT) and mHTT. ASOs are synthetic, short, single-stranded DNA sequences designed to target mRNA. This ASO forms a hybridized complex with RNA that is degraded through an RNAse-H1 mechanism. The clinical trial results suggest that IONIS-HTTRx is safe, well tolerated and is associated with a 40-60% reduction in CSF mHTT concentration at the two highest doses. This reduction may correspond to a 55–85% reduction in cortical mHTT levels (Tabrizi et al. 2019). Currently, two open-label extensions are ongoing (NCT03342053 and NCT03842969) for those who participated in the prior investigational studies. In addition, there is a third active, interventional trial (NCT03761849), which is a phase 3, randomized, double-blind, placebo-controlled study that will evaluate safety and efficacy of RG6042[1] in patients with manifest HD. This pivotal trial will have two primary clinical outcomes for regulatory purposes, the UHDRS TFC score for the FDA, and the composite UHDRS (cUHDRS) for the European Medicines Agency (EMA). Secondary outcomes will involve other components of the UHDRS, clinical global impression, adverse events, cognitive and behavioral assessments, pharmacokinetic markers, CSF levels

---

* IONIS-HTTRx, RO7234292, ISIS 443139 and RG6042 refers to same molecule.

of mTTT and neurofilament light chain, and MRI brain volumes (Rodrigues, Quinn, and Wild 2019).

There are two additional randomized, double-blind, placebo-controlled, phase Ia/IIb trials to study allele-specific ASOs, WVE-120101 (PRECISION-HD1) and WVE-120102 (PRECISION-HD2) (NCT0322 5833 and NCT03225846, respectively). These studies will assess the safety, tolerability, pharmacokinetics, and pharmacodynamics after intrathecal injections in 48 patients with early manifest HD. The allele-selectivity has been achieved by developing stereopure ASOs directed at specific single nucleotide polymorphisms (SNPs). These trials will enroll subjects with specific *HTT* SNPs on the same allele as the pathogenic CAG expansion. Given that HTT is a highly conserved protein with several important cellular functions (Schulte and Littleton 2011), it will be necessary to define the impact of wtHTT reduction in future investigations.

Other strategies to silence or edit HTT were developed in preclinical models and they are promising future approaches for clinical trials in HD. These potential modalities involve the neutralization of targeted mRNA molecules by employing siRNA and artificial microRNA (miRNA), thus inhibiting gene expression or translation, a process known as RNA interference (RNAi) (McBride et al. 2008; DiFiglia et al. 2007). For example, a study showed that adeno-associated viral (AAV) vector designed to deliver siRNA is effective at transducing more than 80% of the cells in the striatum and reducing around 40% of the levels of both wtHTT and mHTT in the same brain region of yeast artificial chromosome (YAC)128 mice. The YAC128 mouse model of HD harbors a mutant human *HTT* gene bearing 128 CAG repeats and exhibits characteristic HD pathology and progressive motor abnormalities. Noteworthy, the authors also described significant improvements in HD-associated behavioral deficits and reduction of striatal HTT aggregates with the AAV-mediated delivery of siRNA in YAC128 mice (Stanek et al. 2014). Another study showed that the treatment with cc-siRNA-HTT (cholesterol-conjugated small interfering RNA duplexes) prolonged survival of striatal neurons, and ameliorated HD-related neuropathology and motor deficits in an acute AAV-mediated transgenic mouse model of HD (created by injecting into the striatum AAV containing 100 CAG HTT cDNA encoding huntingtin 1–400) (DiFiglia et al. 2007). In a study with a transgenic sheep model of HD, AAV delivered artificial miRNA was able to reduce 50-80% of mHTT mRNA and protein in the striatum in addition to no loss of neurons, as evaluated 1 and 6 months post-injection. This study highlighted relevance in demonstrating that effective silencing of mHTT by AAV delivered artificial miRNA can be achieved and sustained in a large-animal brain (Pfister et al. 2018).

Although RNAi and ASOs have been successful in reducing HTT in animal models of HD, the efficacy of these treatments in humans is still a matter of debate, especially because these therapeutic options decrease both wtHTT and mHTT levels. Besides, basal mutant protein levels are still detected. Given the fact that huntingtin is ubiquitously expressed and an important protein for several cellular functions, the use of strategies to direct allele-specific genome editing is an attractive alternative to the partial reduction approach using ASOs or RNAi methods. In this regard, the Clustered Regularly Interspaced Short Palindromic Repeats (CRISPR)/ CRISPR-associated (Cas)9 system has emerged as a promising option, due to its potency and sequence specificity thus mitigating expression from the mutant allele only. Accordingly, CRISP/Cas9 has been regarded as a promising therapy for HD and several other diseases in which DNA editing can be beneficial. The CRISPR/Cas9 system is used by bacterial immune systems in order to cleave foreign DNA. This is a potent and sequence-specific tool for genome editing with a multitude of applications. The CRISPR/Cas9 technology was used in fibroblasts of an HD patient to delete the promoter regions, transcription start site and the CAG mutation expansion of the mutant *HTT* gene, resulting in complete inactivation of the mutant allele without affecting the normal allele (Shin et al. 2016). Recently, this method was successfully tested in an HD rodent model (HD140Q-knockin mice). The CRISPR/Cas9-mediated inactivation efficiently depleted HTT, reversing the HD-associated neuropathology and behavioral phenotypes. The decrease of mHTT expression in striatal neuronal cells in adult HD140Q-knockin mice did not affect cell viability, but alleviated motor deficits (Yang et al. 2017). Despite the positive results obtained from preclinical studies, several issues must be addressed before bringing

CRISPR/Cas9 technologies to clinical trials, especially: i) the fact that it is an irreversible method; ii) there are ethical concerns regarding germline alteration; iii) delivery problems as with other virally delivered approaches; and iv) immunogenicity of bacterial proteins (Tabrizi, Ghosh, and Leavitt 2019).

Anyway, silencing mHTT in the brain continues to be a promising therapeutic strategy for HD. In this regard, a clinical trial is expected to be launched soon to test a new gene therapy product (AM-130) in patients with HD. AM-130 consists of an engineered microRNA targeting human HTT, delivered via adeno-associated viral vector serotype 5 (AAV5-miHTT). One-time intrastriatal administration of AAV5-miHTT in transgenic HD minipigs resulted in a strong, widespread and sustained (up to 12 months) reduction of mHTT levels. The encouraging preclinical results on mutant HTT protein lowering in several brain regions supported the continuation of this program into the clinic. The uniQure trial has therefore been planned and authorized by the FDA and will soon test this therapy (AMT-130) in humans.[1]

HTT Modulation

Strategies targeting the modulation of HTT include its clearance or aggregation inhibition. One study published in 2015 aimed to assess the safety, tolerability, and efficacy of PBT2 in patients with HD. PBT2 is an 8-hydroxyquinoline transition metal ligand that redistributes metals like copper, zinc, and iron from locations where they are abundant to subcellular locations where they might be deficient (Huntington Study Group Reach 2015). Excessive metal concentrations induce mHTT aggregation and promote formation of reactive oxygen species (ROS). Therefore, it has been hypothesized that PBT2 could attenuate mHTT effects by inhibiting metal-induced aggregation of mHTT and ROS formation. Accordingly, PBT2 has been effective in ameliorating the HD phenotype in both *C. elegans* and R6/2

---

[1] http://uniqure.com/gene-therapy/huntingtons-disease.php

mice models of HD (Cherny et al. 2012). The clinical trial (NCT01590888) was designed as a 26-week, phase II, randomized, double-blind, placebo-controlled study and 109 participants were randomly assigned to PBT2 250 mg, PBT2 100 mg, or placebo. In the end, 89% of individuals on PBT2 250 mg, 100% on PBT2 100 mg, and 97% on placebo completed the study. Several adverse events occurred in participants receiving PBT2. However, the investigators deemed all but one (worsening of HD) as unrelated with PBT2. A significant improvement was observed in one measure of executive function (Trail Making Test Part B score) in the 250 mg group, but this isolated finding is of limited clinical relevance. Of note, the overall cognitive composite measured was not improved (Huntington Study Group Reach 2015). Overall, PBT2 was considered safe and well-tolerated; however, the US Food and Drug Administration (FDA) issued a Partial Clinical Hold in 2015 due to safety concerns of the 250 mg dose and required more neurotoxicity data for the continuity of clinical trials with PBT2. There have been no recent updates.

Another study focusing on promotion of the HTT clearance was performed using selisistat, a SirT1 (silent information regulator T1) inhibitor, first-in-class, for which an exact mechanism of action has not been established (La Spada, Weydt, and Pineda 2011). SirT1 is a member of the sirtuin deacetylase family and one of few that can remove acetyl groups from mHTT. Inhibition of SirT1 in Drosophila and mouse models of HD resulted in a selective decrease of mHTT levels (Pallos et al. 2008; M.R. Smith et al. 2014). Selisistat (SEN0014196) has been tested in two double-blind, placebo-controlled clinical trials focused primarily in safety and tolerability assessing a short-term (NCT01485952, 14 days) (Sussmuth et al. 2015) and a long-term (NCT01521585, 12 weeks) treatment duration (R. Reilmann et al. 2014). Although both studies have demonstrated that selisitat is safe and well-tolerated, they failed to show significant differences between selisistat and placebo groups in terms of efficacy and other outcomes that included motor and cognition symptoms, and functional capacity. Another trail has been registered (NCT01485965) aiming at assessing fasted *vs.* fed conditions, i.e., the effect of food on the pharmacokinetics of SEN0014196 in patients with HD. The study was designed explore potential biomarkers for use in subsequent Phase 2/3 studies, but no results have been published so far. Currently, there are no phase III trials planned, and further development appears to be on hold.

Immunomodulatory Therapies

Immune dysregulation has been implicated in pathogeneses of HD. Accordingly, the immune system has been a target for clinical trials of HD-modifying therapies. Laquinimod is an immunomodulatory drug originally studied for the treatment of relapsing-remitting multiple sclerosis (Thone et al. 2012; Comi et al. 2012). The precise mechanism of action is still unknown but some hypotheses include the inhibition of astrocyte activation, restoration of brain-derived neurotrophic factor (BDNF) levels, and modulation of the mitogen-activated protein kinase (MAPK) signaling pathway (Wild and Tabrizi 2014). In mouse models of HD, laquinimod treatment decreased the levels of pro-apoptotic proteins, reduced interleukin (IL)-6 levels and improved behavior related to motor and psychiatric symptoms (Ehrnhoefer et al. 2016; Garcia-Miralles et al. 2016). A clinical trial was then conducted with patients with HD. The LEGATO-HD is a phase 2, 12-month, multicenter, randomized, placebo-controlled, double-blind trial using the laquinimod 0.5 and 1.0 mg/day (NCT02215616)*. After one year, the laquinomod treatment resulted in no changes in the Unified Huntington Disease Rating Scale (UHDRS) score, as compared with placebo. However, the laquinimod treatment resulted a significant reduction of caudate atrophy and whole brain atrophy that was most evident in early HD patients (Biotech 2019). At this time, it is unclear how a positive imaging-based secondary outcome in the setting of a negative clinical primary outcome should be interpreted. One hypothesis is that the treatment would be more efficient if initiated years (or even decades) before the disease onset, thus preventing neurodegeneration. More data is required to understand the significance of these results.

---

* The original Legato-HD protocol included the treatment with 1.5 mg of laquinimod, but this dose arm was discontinued later as a proactive safety measure.

Table 1. Past clinical trials in Huntington's disease registered at ClinicalTrials.gov

Huntingtin (HTT)-lowering and HTT modulation therapies

Study Title	Phase/Design	Registration ID	S or DM	Intervention/ Treatment	N	Study Status/Results
Safety, Tolerability, Pharmacokinetics, and Pharmacodynamics of ISIS 443139 in Participants With Early Manifest Huntington's Disease (IONIS-HTTRx).	Phase 1/2a; 13-week randomized, double-blind, placebo-controlled study.	NCT02519036	DM	Intrathecal injections of ISIS 443139 aka IONIS-HTTRx (10, 30, 60, 90, 120 mg) every 4 weeks.	46	Completed. No serious adverse events were reported. There was a dose-dependent reduction in the concentration of mutant huntingtin in CSF (Tabrizi et al. 2019).
Effect of PBT2 in Patients With Early to Mid-Stage Huntington Disease (Reach2HD).	Phase 2; 26-week, randomized, double-blind, placebo-controlled trial.	NCT01590888	DM	PBT2 100 or 250 mg daily.	109	Completed. PBT2 was well tolerated and safe. There was an improvement in the performance on a scale evaluating executive function with PBT2 250 mg compared with placebo (Huntington Study Group Reach 2015).
An Exploratory Clinical Trial in Early Stage Huntington's Disease Patients With SEN0014196 (PADDINGTON).	Phase 1; 14-day, randomized, double-blind, placebo-controlled, parallel-assignment study.	NCT01485952	DM	SEN0014196 (Selisistat) 10 or 100 mg, once a day.	55	Completed. Selisistat was found to be safe and well tolerated in early stage HD patients at plasma concentrations providing benefit in non-clinical HD models (Sussmuth et al. 2015).
A Phase II Safety and Tolerability Study With SEN0014196.	Phase 2; 12-week, randomized, double-blind, placebo-controlled study.	NCT01521585	DM	SEN0014196 (Selisistat) 50 or 200 mg, once a day.	144	Completed. Selisistat was safe and well tolerated, and there was a trend for modulation of blood levels of soluble mutant huntingtin (R.Reilmann et al. 2014).
An Open-label Food Effect Study With SEN0014196 in Subjects With Huntington Disease.	Phase 1b, 14-day, open-label, parallel-group (fasted vs. fed conditions) study.	NCT01485965	DM	SEN0014196 (Selisistat) 100 mg once a day.	26	Completed. No results found.
Effects of EGCG (Epigallocatechin Gallate) in Huntington's Disease (ETON-Study) (ETON).	Phase 2; 12-month, randomized, placebo-controlled, double-blind study.	NCT01357681	DM/S	(2)-epigallocatechin-3-gallate (EGCG) up to 1200 mg.	54	Completed. No results were found.

Study Title	Phase/Design	Registration ID	S or DM	Intervention/ Treatment	N	Study Status/Results
Immunomodulatory/anti-inflammatory therapies						
A Clinical Study in Participants With Huntington's Disease (HD) to Assess Efficacy and Safety of Three Oral Doses of Laquinimod (LEGATO-HD).	Phase 2; 12-month randomized, double-blind, placebo-controlled, parallel-group study.	NCT02215616	DM/S	Laquinimod 0.5, 1.0 and 1.5 mg/Day	352	Completed. No changes in the UHDRS score, but a significant reduction of caudate atrophy and whole brain atrophy that was most evident in early HD patients (press release).
Minocycline in Patients With Huntington's Disease.	Phase 1/2; 8-week, double-blind, randomized, placebo-controlled study.	NCT00029874	DM/S	Minocycline 100 or 200 mg/day	60	Completed. Minocycline was well tolerated, but no efficacy was observed (no effect on the UHDRS or cognitive tests scores)(Huntington Study Group 2004).
Pilot Study of Minocycline in Huntington's Disease.	Phase 2/3;18-month, randomized, double-blind, placebo-controlled, parallel-group study	NCT00277355	DM/S	Minocycline 100 mg twice a day (200 mg/day)	114	Completed. Minocycline was well tolerated and safe. The small decline in TFC score in the minocycline group suggested futility; the results provides insufficient evidence to justify a larger and longer trial of minocycline in HD (D.I. Huntington Study Group 2010).
Study Exploring Safety, Pharmacokinetic and Pharmacodynamic of BN82451 in Male Huntington's Disease Patients	Phase 2a; 4-week, randomized, placebo-controlled, parallel assignment study.	NCT02231580	S/DM	BN82451B 40-80 mg twice daily.	17	Terminated prematurely due to subject recruitment issues.
Metabolic- and mitochondrial-based protective strategies						
Coenzyme Q10 in Huntington's Disease (HD) (2CARE).	Phase 3; 60-month, randomized, double-blind, placebo-controlled trial	NCT0060881	DM	Coenzyme Q10 (CoQ10) 240 mg/day.	609	Terminated. CoQ10 was generally safe and well tolerated. A futility analysis failed to show likelihood of benefit of CoQ10 2400 mg/day (McGarry, McDermott, et al. 2017).
Study in PRE-manifest Huntington's Disease of Coenzyme Q10 (UbiquinonE) Leading to Preventive Trials (PREQUEL).	Phase 2; 20-week, randomized, double-blind, parallel group study.	NCT00920699	DM	Coenzyme Q10 (CoQ10) 600, 1200, 2400 mg per day.	90	Completed. CoQ10 was generally safe and well tolerated. CoQ10 treatment was associated with increases in serum levels of CoQ10, but with no change in 8OHdG levels. There was no relationship between 8OHdG level and predicted age of disease onset (C. Ross, Biglan, et al. 2014; Biglan et al. 2014).

Table 1. (Continued)

Study Title	Phase/Design	Registration ID	S or DM	Intervention/ Treatment	N	Study Status/Results
Metabolic- and mitochondrial-based protective strategies						
Bioavailability of Ubiquinol in Huntington Disease.	Phase 1; 8-week, open-label, single group assignment study.	NCT00980694	DM	Ubiquinol (Coenzyme Q10) up to 600mg a day	6	Completed. No results have been published.
Creatine Therapy for Huntington's Disease (CREST-HD).	Phase 1/2; 16-week, randomized, double-blind, placebo-controlled study.	NCT00026988	DM	Creatine 8g daily.	64	Completed. Creatine 8g/day was well tolerated and safe. Serum and brain creatine concentrations increased in the creatine-treated group and returned to baseline after washout. Serum 8-hydroxy-2'-deoxyguanosine levels, an indicator of oxidative injury to DNA, were markedly elevated in HD and reduced by creatine treatment. Clinical measures were unchanged over the treatment course (UHDRS) (S.M. Hersch et al. 2006).
Creatine Safety and Tolerability in Premanifest HD (PRECREST).	Phase 2; randomized, placebo-controlled, 18-month (6-month double-blind phase followed by a 12-month open-label extension) study.	NCT00592995	DM	Creatine monohydrate 30 g daily.	64	Completed. Creatine was well tolerated and safe. Neuroimaging demonstrated treatment-related slowing of cortical and striatal atrophy at 6 and 18 months. No improvement in clinical symptoms (Rosas et al. 2014).
Premanifest Huntington's Disease: Creatine Safety & Tolerability Extension Study (PRECREST-X).	Phase 2; 12-month, open-label, single group assignment study.	NCT01411150	DM	Creatine monohydrate 30 g daily.	38	Completed. Open-label extension of the PRE-CREST study. Creatine was well tolerated and safe. Neuroimaging demonstrated treatment-related slowing of cortical and striatal atrophy at 6 and 18 months. No improvement in clinical symptoms (Rosas et al. 2014).
Premanifest Huntington's Disease Extension Study II: Creatine Safety & Tolerability (PRECREST-2X).	Phase 2; 24-month, open-label, single group assignment study.	NCT01411163	DM	Creatine Monohydrate (up to 30 g)	24	Completed. No results have been published. The purpose of this clinical trial was to extend the PreCrest-X to further assess the long-term safety and tolerability.

Study Title	Phase/Design	Registration ID	S or DM	Intervention /Treatment	N	Study Status/Results
Metabolic- and mitochondrial-based protective strategies						
Creatine Safety & Tolerability in Huntington's Disease (CREST-X).	Phase 2; open-label, long-term safety & tolerability extension study (44 months) of creatine in subjects with HD	NCT01412151	DM	Creatine Monohydrate up to 30 g daily	10	Completed. Creatine is well tolerated and safe in patients with HD.
Creatine Safety, Tolerability, & Efficacy in Huntington's Disease (CREST-E).	Phase 3; randomized, placebo-controlled, 48-month study.	NCT00712426	DM	Creatine monohydrate up to 40 g daily	553	Terminated because results of an interim analysis showed a lack of promise for creatine in slowing disease progression in patients with early-HD (S.M. Hersch et al. 2017).
Study Evaluating The Safety, Tolerability And Brain Function Of 2 Doses Of PF-0254920 In Subjects With Early Huntington's Disease.	Phase 2; 28-day, randomized, double-blind, placebo-controlled study.	NCT01806896	DM	PF-02545920 5 or 20 mg twice a day.	37	Completed. PF-02545920 was generally safe tolerated. Patients receiving PF-02545920 showed a significant improvement in their physical effort in response to incentive motivation during a grip-strength test.
Randomized, Placebo Controlled Study Of The Efficacy And Safety Of PF-02545920 In Subjects With Huntington's Disease (Amaryllis trial).	Phase 2; 26-week, randomized, double-blind, placebo-controlled, parallel assignment study.	NCT02197130	DM/S	PF-02545920 5 or 20 mg twice a day.	272	Completed. PF-02545920 was generally safe tolerated: adverse events were generally mild or moderate and occurred more frequently at 20mg. There was no evidence of efficacy in primary (change in UHDRS-TMS score) or secondary clinical endpoints with PF02545920 5 mg or 20 mg BID (M. Delnomdedieu et al. 2018).
Open Label Extension Study To Investigate Long Term Safety, Tolerability And Efficacy Of PF-02545920 In Subjects With Huntington's Disease Who Completed Study A8241021 (NCT02197130)	Phase 2, 12-month open-label extension of NCT02197130	NCT02342548	DM/S	PF-02545920 20mg twice a day.	188	Terminated because the results from the previous study (NCT02197130) did not meet pre-defined efficacy criteria for improvement of motor symptoms and many of the secondary assessments (TMC and CGI-I scores) were not significantly different from baseline (M.Delnomdedieu 2018).
TREND-HD - A Trial of Ethyl-EPA (Miraxion™) in Treating	Phase 3; 6-month, randomized, double-	NCT00146211	DM/S	Ethyl-EPA (Miraxion™) 2 gram per day.	316	Completed. Ethyl-EPA was not beneficial. No differences were found in measures of

Table 1. (Continued)

Study Title	Phase/Design	Registration ID	S or DM	Intervention/ Treatment	N	Study Status/Results
Metabolic- and mitochondrial-based protective strategies						
Mild to Moderate Huntington's Disease.	blind, placebo-controlled study.					motor function, global functioning cognition, or global impression (Huntington Study Group 2008).
Proof of Concept of an Anaplerotic Study Using Brain Phosphorus Magnetic Resonance Spectroscopy in Huntington Disease (TRIHEP2).	Phase 2; 1-month, open-label, single-group assignment study.	NCT01882062	DM	Triheptanoin 1g/kg body weight/day	10	Completed. Triheptanoin was shown to correct the brain bioenergetic profile (based on the inorganic phosphate /phosphocreatine ratio) in early stage HD (Adanyeguh et al. 2015).
Safety Study of the Novel Drug Dimebon to Treat Patients With Huntington's Disease.	Phase 1/2; 7-day, randomized, open-label, dosage-escalation, placebo-controlled study.	NCT00387270	DM/S	Dimebon (latrepirdine) 10 or 20 mg 3 times a day.	9	Completed. No results found.
A Study of the Novel Drug Dimebon in Patients With Huntington's Disease (DIMOND).	Phase 2; 3-month, randomized, double-blind, placebo-controlled trial.	NCT00497159	DM/S	Dimebon (latrepirdine) 20 mg 3 times a day.	91	Completed. Latrepirdine was well tolerated and showed a discrete but significant improvement in one of the cognitive scales (MMSE). No significant treatment effects were seen on the UHDRS or the ADAS-cog (Kieburtz et al. 2010).
A Safety and Efficacy Study of Dimebon in Patients With Huntington Disease (HORIZON).	Phase 3; 26-week, randomized, double-blind, placebo-controlled study.	NCT00920946	DM/S	Dimebon (latrepirdine) 20 mg 3 times a day.	403	Completed. Latrepirdine was safe and well tolerated but did not improve cognition or global function in patients with HD with baseline cognitive impairment (Horizon Investigators of the Huntington Study Group and European Huntington's Disease Network 2013).
An Extension of the HORIZON Protocol Evaluating the Safety of Dimebon (Latrepirdine) in Subjects With Huntington Disease (HORIZON PLUS).	Phase 3; single-group assignment, open-label extension of the HORIZON protocol.	NCT01085266	DM/S	Dimebon (latrepirdine) 20 mg 3 times a day.	362	Terminated because of the unsuccessful HORIZON trial (NCT00920946) results.

Study Title	Phase/Design	Registration ID	S or DM	Intervention /Treatment	N	Study Status/Results
Metabolic- and mitochondrial-based protective strategies						
Safety and Efficacy of OMS643762 in Subjects With Huntington's Disease	Phase 2; 4-week, randomized, double-blind, placebo-controlled, parallel assignment study.	NCT02074410	DM/S	OMS643762	22	Terminated per sponsor decision - pending further analysis of available data.
Other disease-modifying therapies						
Neuroprotection by Cannabinoids in Huntington's Disease.	Phase 2; 12-week, randomized, double-blind, placebo-controlled, crossover pilot.	NCT01502046	DM/S	Sativex(®) [delta-9-tetrahydrocannabinol (THC) + cannabidiol (CBD)] 12 sprays/day.	25	Completed. Safety and tolerability were confirmed. No differences on motor, cognitive, behavioral and functional scores were detected as compared to placebo (Lopez-Sendon Moreno et al. 2016).
Safety and Tolerability Study of Phenylbutyrate in Huntington's Disease (PHEND-HD).	Phase 2; one-month, randomized, placebo-controlled study, followed by a 12-week open-label treatment.	NCT00212316	DM/S	Sodium phenylbutyrate 15 g daily.	60	Completed. Phenylbutyrate was safe and well tolerated in early symptomatic HD subjects (S. Hersch and Huntington Study Group 2008).
Riluzole in Huntington's Disease.	Phase 3; 3-year, randomized, double-blind, placebo-controlled study.	NCT00277602	DM/S	Riluzole 50 mg twice daily.	537	Completed. No neuroprotective or beneficial symptomatic effects of riluzole were demonstrated (Landwehrmeyer et al. 2007).
MIG-HD: Multicentric Intracerebral Grafting in Huntington's Disease (MIG-HD).	Phase 2; 52-month, randomized, open-label, parallel assignment (grafted vs. not yet grafted patients) study.	NCT00190450	DM	Intrastriatal grafting of human cells from the fetal ganglionic eminence	54	Completed. The results of MIG-HD are not yet available. The trial has demonstrated that immunosuppression is required and has established a new surgical procedure to avoid subdural hematoma (Bachoud-Levi 2017).
Effects of Lithium and Divalproex on Brain-Derived Neurotrophic Factor in Huntington's Disease.	Phase 2, 6-week, placebo-controlled study.	NCT00095355	DM	Lithium carbonate alone or with divalproex.	35	Completed. No results were found
Symptomatic treatments						
Neuroleptic and Huntington Disease Comparison of: Olanzapine, la Tetrabenazine and Tiapride (NEUROHD)	Phase 3; 12-month, randomized, single-group assignment, open-label study.	NCT00632645	S	Olanzapine 2.5-20 mg per day, Xenazine 25-200 mg per day, and Tiapridal 300-800 mg per day.	180	Completed. No results found.

Table 1. (Continued)

Study Title	Phase/Design	Registration ID	S or DM	Intervention/ Treatment	N	Study Status/Results
Symptomatic treatments						
Atomoxetine and Huntington's Disease.	Phase 2; 10-week, randomized, double-blind, placebo-controlled study.	NCT00368849	S	Atomoxetine (Strattera) 80 mg per day.	20	Completed. Atomoxetine was generally well tolerated but demonstrated no advantages over placebo in attention, psychiatric, and motor symptom scores (Beglinger et al. 2009).
Citalopram to Enhance Cognition in HD (CIT-HD)	Phase 2; 20-week, randomized, placebo-controlled pilot study.	NCT00271596	S	Citalopram 20 mg daily.	33	Completed. No evidence that short-term treatment with citalopram improved executive functions. Citalopram improved mood in non-depressed patients (patients with active depression were not included in the study), thus raising the possibility of efficacy for subsyndromal depression in HD (Beglinger et al. 2014).
Apathy Cure Through Bupropion in Huntington's Disease (Action-HD).	Phase 2; 10-week, randomized, double-blind, placebo-controlled, crossover study.	NCT01914965	S	Bupropion 300 mg daily.	40	Completed. Bupropion does not alleviate apathy in HD. Study participation improved symptoms of apathy, regardless of whether the drug or the placebo was administered (Gelderblom et al. 2017).
Efficacy and Safety of Tetrabenazine in Chorea.	Phase 3; 12-week, randomized, double-blind, placebo-controlled study.	NCT00219804	S	Tetrabenazine (TBZ) up to 100mg/day.	84	Completed. TBZ significantly reduced chorea burden, improved global outcome, and was generally safe and well tolerated in the 12-week double-blind study (Huntington Study Group 2006). In the open-label extension study, TBZ continued to effectively suppress chorea for up to 80 weeks and was generally well tolerated (Frank 2009).
Effect of Tetrabenazine on Stroop Interference in HD.	Phase 4; single-group assignment, open-label study.	NCT01834911	S	Tetrabenazine (TBZ) withdrawal	10	Completed. There was a significant deterioration in Stroop Color-Word scores after TBZ withdrawal (Fekete, Davidson, and Jankovic 2012).

Study Title	Phase/Design	Registration ID	S or DM	Intervention/ Treatment	N	Study Status/Results
Symptomatic treatments						
Impact of Xenazine (Tetrabenazine) on Gait and Functional Activity in Individuals With Huntington's Disease.	Single-group assignment, open-label study.	NCT01451463		Tetrabenazine (TBZ) withdrawal	11	Completed. TBZ use may improve balance and functional mobility in individuals with HD (Kegelmeyer et al. 2014).
First Time Use of SD-809 in Huntington Disease (First-HD)	Phase 3; 12-week, randomized double-blind, placebo-controlled study.	NCT01795859	S	SD-809 (deutetrabenazine) 6-48 mg per day.	90	Completed. Deutetrabenazine treatment significantly improved chorea control together with improvements in patient-centered end-points in comparison with placebo (Huntington Study Group et al. 2016).
Alternatives for Reducing Chorea in Huntington Disease (ARC-HD)	Phase 3; non-randomized, single-group assignment, open-label, long term safety study [for participants who completed First-HD (NCT01795859) or participants who were receiving FDA - approved dosing regimen of tetrabenazine.	NCT01897896	S	SD-809 (deutetrabenazine) Initial daily dose: 6-48mg	119	Completed. Safety and tolerability of deutetrabenazine was comparable to that of tetrabenazine. The overnight conversion to deutetrabenazine therapy provided a favorable safety profile and effectively maintained chorea control (Frank et al. 2017).
A Study of Treatment With Pridopidine (ACR16) in Patients With Huntington's Disease (MermaiHD).	Phase 3; 6-month, randomized, double-blind, placebo-controlled, parallel group study	NCT00665223	S	Pridopidine (ACR 16) 22.5 or 45 mg twice a day.	437	Completed. Pridopidine was well tolerated and the 90mg/day dose had a potential effect on motor abilities (de Yebenes et al. 2011).
A Study of Pridopidine (ACR16) for the Treatment of Patients With Huntington's Disease (HART)	Phase 2/3; 12-week, randomized, double-blind, placebo-controlled, parallel group study.	NCT00724048	S	Pridopidine (ACR16) 10, 22.5, and 45 mg twice a day.	227	Completed. Pridopidine was generally well tolerated. Although not statistically significant, the overall results suggested an improvement in motor function with the 90 mg/day dosage (H.I. Huntington Study Group 2013).

Table 1. (Continued)

Study Title	Phase/Design	Registration ID	S or DM	Intervention/ Treatment	N	Study Status/Results
Symptomatic treatments						
Open-label Extension Study of Pridopidine (ACR16) in the Symptomatic Treatment of Huntington Disease (OPEN-HART)	Phase 2; 36-month, open-label, single group assignment study.	NCT01306929	S	Pridopidine 45 mg twice a day.	235	Completed. Pridopidine 45 mg taken twice a day was generally safe and tolerable. Patients progressed according to generally accepted trends of the disease (McGarry, Kieburtz, et al. 2017).
A Phase 2, to Evaluating the Safety and Efficacy of Pridopidine Versus Placebo for Symptomatic Treatment in Patients With Huntington's Disease (PRIDE-HD)	Phase 2; 52-week, randomized, double-blind, placebo-controlled, dose range finding study.	NCT02006472	S	Pridopidine 45, 67.5, 90, and 112.5 mg twice a day.	408	Completed. At week 26, pridopidine did not improve the patients' total motor score. Serious adverse effects and one death were reported in the treatment group only, as well as a strong placebo effect (R. Reilmann et al. 2019).
A Study Evaluating if Pridopidine is Safe, Efficacious, and Tolerable in Patients With Huntington's Disease (Open PRIDE-HD)	Phase 2; single-group assignment, open-label study.	NCT02494778	S	Pridopidine 45 mg twice daily.	248	Terminated. The study served its purpose in providing safety data. Termination was not associated with any new or emerging safety concern.
Treatment of Huntington's Chorea With Amantadine	Phase2; 2-week, randomized, placebo-controlled, crossover trial.	NCT00001930	S	Amantadine 100 mg 3 times daily.	24	Completed. Amantadine was not effective for HD chorea, although most patients felt subjectively better during the amantadine treatment (O'Suilleabhain and Dewey 2003).
A Trial of Memantine as Symptomatic Treatment for Early Huntington Disease (MITIGATE-HD).	Phase 2b; 24-week, randomized, double-blind, placebo-controlled study.	NCT01458470	S	Memantine 10 mg twice daily.	19	Completed. No results published yet.
Efficacy, Safety and Tolerability of AFQ056 in Patients With Huntington's Disease in Reducing Chorea	Phase 2; 32-day randomized, double-blind, placebo-controlled, parallel-group study.	NCT01019473	S	AFQ056 (mavoglurant) 25-150 mg twice a day.	44	Terminated. AFQ056 was well tolerated but did not reduce chorea in HD. AFQ056 may reduce variability of finger taps (R. Reilmann et al. 2015).
Tolerability, Safety, and Activity of SRX246 in Irritable Subjects With Huntington's Disease.	Phase 1/2; 12-week, randomized, double-blind,	NCT02507284	S	SRX246 120 mg and 160 mg twice a day.	106	Completed. The results have not been published yet.

Study Title	Phase/Design	Registration ID	S or DM	Intervention/ Treatment	N	Study Status/Results
Symptomatic treatments						
	placebo-controlled, factorial assignment study.					
Treating Sleep/Wake Cycle Disturbances in Basal Ganglia Disorders With Ramelteon.	Randomized, double-blind, placebo-controlled, pilot study.	NCT00907595	S	Ramelteon	0	Withdrawn. The investigators were unable to recruit subjects.
Non-pharmacological treatments						
Working Memory Training in Huntington's Disease.	Phase 1/2; 25-session, single group assignment.	NCT02926820	S	Cogmed (computerized cognitive training) 5 days/week for 5 weeks.	9	Completed. 7/9 participants adhered to training; all 7 showed improvement on the Cogmed tasks and reported that they found training helpful. Adherent participants also reported that it was difficult, frustrating, and time-consuming (Sadeghi et al. 2017).
Exploring Computerised Cognitive Training for People With Huntington's Disease (CogTrainHD).	12-week, randomized, open-label, parallel assignment study.	NCT02990676	S	CogTrainHD (computerized cognitive training).	30	Completed. No results published yet. This study aimed to assess the feasibility of delivering a home-based computerized cognitive training for people with HD (Yhnell et al. 2018).
Effects of Music Therapy on Huntington's Disease.	Phase 1; 6-week, randomized, crossover assignment study.	NCT00178360	S	Music Therapy; one individual and one group session per week.	5	Completed. Music therapy was well tolerated. There was improvement in UHDRS scores for finger tapping, pronation/supination, and the Luria, but the changes did not achieve statistical significance with the small sample size in this study (Hyson et al. 2005).
Laughter Therapy Effects on Mood, Stress and Self-efficacy in People With Neurological Diseases.	Non-randomized, open-label, single-group assignment study.	NCT02750982	S	60-minute laughter therapy, 8 sessions.	24	Completed. No results published yet.
The Effect of Video Game Exercise on Dynamic Balance and Gait in Individuals With Huntington's Disease.	Crossover, controlled, single-blinded, six-week trial.	NCT01735981	S	45-minute supervised program using *Dance Dance Revolution* or unsupervised handheld game, twice a week.	18	Completed. The intervention was safe, feasible and motivating. Significant changes were noted in dynamic balance during walking. No significant impact on functional mobility, balance confidence, or quality of life (Kloos et al. 2013).

Table 1. (Continued)

Study Title	Phase/Design	Registration ID	S or DM	Intervention/ Treatment	N	Study Status/Results
Non-pharmacological treatments						
Treadmill Walking in Individuals With Dementia With Lewy Bodies and Huntington's Disease.	Non-randomized, open-label, single-group assignment study.	NCT02268617	S	20-minute session treadmill walking	28	Completed. No results were found.
Dance and Huntington Disease.	5-month, non-randomized, parallel assignment (standard care vs. experimental group) study.	NCT01842919	S	Contemporary dance training practiced for two hours per week.	19	Completed. Adherence was very good. The practice improved motor function along with increased brain volume in areas supporting spatial and somatosensory processing. There were no changes in cognitive or behavioral measures (Trinkler et al. 2019).
Exercise Effects in Huntington's Disease.	26-week, non-randomized, parallel assignment (HD vs. healthy controls) study.	NCT01879267	DM/S	Endurance training.	40	Completed. Endurance training was safe and feasible. The training enhanced indices of energy metabolism in skeletal muscle, being a potential therapeutic approach to delay the onset and/or progression of muscular dysfunction in HD (Mueller et al. 2017).
Feasibility and Acceptability of Implementing a Clinic-based Physical Activity Coaching Intervention in People With Premanifest and Early Stage HD	Phase 1/2; 4-month, open-label, single group assignment study.	NCT03306888	S	One one-hour face-to-face coaching session and three 20-minute remote video sessions.	14	Completed. No results published yet.
Electronic-health Application To Measure Outcomes REmotely Clinical Trial (EAT MORE)	6-month, randomized open-label, standard-of-care-controlled study.	NCT02418546	S	Nutritional Counseling (in-person by registered dietician or online using an E-Health application).	88	Completed. Results were recently published for patients with amyotrophic lateral sclerosis. Nutritional counseling by a registered dietitian (with or without support by an app) is safe but did not maintain weight significantly better than standard care (Wills et al. 2019).
Deep Brain Stimulation of the Globus Pallidus in Huntington's Disease.	Phase 1, 6-month, randomized, double-blind, controlled, crossover [stimulation	NCT00902889	S	Deep Brain Stimulation (DBS)	6	Completed. DBS electrode implantation can be performed in a safe procedure. GPE stimulation was equivalent to GPI stimulation; chronic stimulation of the

Study Title	Phase/Design	Registration ID	S or DM	Intervention/ Treatment	N	Study Status/Results
	of the external pallidum (GPE) vs. internal pallidum (GPI)] study.					pallidum significant reduced chorea; effects on dystonic symptoms varied inter-individually from no response to a strong response. Hypokinetic-rigid symptoms and Westphal patients did not improve. Cognition was generally stable. Several measures of quality of life and functionality improved significantly, as did measures of mood (Wojtecki et al. 2015).
The Effect of tDCS on Subcortical Brain Functioning.	Randomized, crossover assignment.	NCT01602276	S	Transcranial Direct Current Stimulation (tDCS)	3	Terminated. Terminated because of problems finding appropriate patients.
Walking While Talking: The Effect of Doing Two Things at Once in Individuals With Neurological Injury or Disease	Non-randomized, open-label, single-group assignment study.	NCT01917903	S	Gait-cognitive training and Identification of at risk variables	100	Suspended because funding ended.

S = Symptomatic and DM = disease-modifying treatment.

Table 2. Current/future trials in Huntington's disease registered at ClinicalTrials.gov

Study Title	Phase/Design	Registration ID	S or DM	Intervention/ Treatment	N	Study Status/Results
Disease-modifying treatments						
A Study to Evaluate the Safety, Tolerability, Pharmacokinetics, and Pharmacodynamics of RO7234292 (ISIS 443139) in Huntington's Disease Patients Who Participated in Prior Investigational Studies of RO7234292 (ISIS 443139).	Phase 2; 14-month, open-label extension study. **Active, not recruiting.**	NCT03342053	S/DM	RO7234292 (RG6042, ISIS 443139 or IONIS-HTTRx)	46	This study will evaluate the safety, tolerability, pharmacokinetics/ pharmacodynamics and efficacy of RO7234292 in patients with HD who previously participated in the IONIS-HTTRx trial (NCT02519036).
An Open-Label Extension Study to Evaluate Long-Term Safety and Tolerability of RO7234292 (RG6042) in Huntington's Disease Patients Who Participated in Prior Roche and Genentech Sponsored Studies.	Phase 3; 5-year, open-label extension study. **Recruiting.**	NCT03842969	S/DM	RO7234292 (RG6042, ISIS 443139 or IONIS-HTTRx)	950	This study evaluates the long-term safety/tolerability of RO7234292 (RG6042) in patients with HD who participated in prior Roche and Genentech sponsored studies.

Table 2. (Continued)

Study Title	Phase/Design	Registration ID	S or DM	Intervention/ Treatment	N	Study Status/Results
Disease-modifying treatments						
A Study to Evaluate the Efficacy and Safety of Intrathecally Administered RO7234292 (RG6042) in Patients With Manifest Huntington's Disease.	Phase 3, randomized, double-blind, placebo-controlled study. **Recruiting**	NCT03761849	S/DM	RO7234292 (RG6042).	660	This study will evaluate the efficacy and safety of intrathecally administered RO7234292 (RG6042) in patients with manifest HD.
A Study in Subjects With Late Prodromal and Early Manifest Huntington's Disease (HD) to Assess the Safety, Tolerability, Pharmacokinetics, and Efficacy of Pepinemab (VX15/2503) (SIGNAL).	Phase 2; randomized, double-blind, placebo controlled study. **Active, not recruiting.**	NCT02481674	S/DM	VX15/2503	301	This study will evaluate safety, tolerability, and immunogenicity of VX15/2503 in patients with prodromal and early manifest HD. In addition, the investigators will assess the effect of VX15/2503 on brain volume, clinical symptoms and inflammatory parameters.
Safety and Tolerability of WVE-120101 in Patients With Huntington's Disease (PRECISION-HD1).	Phase 1b/2a; randomized, double-blind, placebo-controlled study. **Recruiting.**	NCT03225833		WVE-120101.	48	PRECISION-HD1 will evaluate the safety, tolerability, pharmacokinetics, and pharmacodynamics of single and multiple doses of WVE-120101 in adult patients with early manifest HD who carry a targeted single nucleotide polymorphism rs362307 (SNP1).
Safety and Tolerability of WVE-120102 in Patients With Huntington's Disease (PRECISION-HD2).	Phase 1b/2a; randomized, double-blind, placebo-controlled study. **Recruiting.**	NCT03225846	S/DM	WVE-120102.	48	PRECISION-HD1 will evaluate the safety, tolerability, pharmacokinetics, and pharmacodynamics of single and multiple doses of WVE-120102 in adult patients with early manifest HD who carry a targeted single nucleotide polymorphism rs362331 (SNP2).
Safety Evaluation of Cellavita HD Administered Intravenously in Participants With Huntington's Disease (SAVE-DH).	Phase 1, non-randomized, open-label study. **Active, not recruiting.**	NCT02728115	DM	Cellavita HD – stem-cell therapy (1x10^6 cells/kg or 2x10^6 cells/kg).	6	This study will evaluate the safety, tolerability, and efficacy of the Cellavita stem cell therapy, administered intravenously. Patients with HD will receive three intravenous injections and will be followed for 5 years to evaluate

Study Title	Phase/Design	Registration ID	S or DM	Intervention/ Treatment	N	Study Status/Results
Disease-modifying treatments						
						safety and tolerability of product and preliminary evidence of effectiveness.
Dose-response Evaluation of the Cellavita HD Product in Patients With Huntington's Disease (ADORE-DH).	Phase 2; randomized, double-blind, placebo-controlled study. **Recruiting**	NCT03252535	DM	Cellavita HD – stem-cell therapy (1x10^6 cells/kg or 2x10^6 cells/kg).	35	This is a phase II dose-response study in which participants with HD will receive three intravenous injections of stem-cell therapy (Cellavita) or placebo (one every month for three months), three cycles.
Resveratrol and Huntington Disease (REVHD).	Randomized, 12-month, double-blind, controlled study. **Active, not recruiting.**	NCT02336633	DM	Resveratrol 80 mg.	102	This study will test the effectiveness of resveratrol in slowing HD progression, as measured by caudate atrophy, and scales assessing motor control, cognitive symptoms, behavioral symptoms, independence, and functioning.
A Comparative Phase 2 Study Assessing the Efficacy of Triheptanoin, an Anaplerotic Therapy in Huntington's Disease (TRIHEP3).	Phase 2; 6-month, randomized, double-blind, controlled study. **Active, not recruiting.**	NCT02453061	DM	Triheptanoin oil 1g/kg/day.	100	This study will evaluate the effect of triheptanoin oil on brain energy restoration and caudate atrophy. Secondary outcomes include motor, cognitive, behavior and functionality measures, in addition to safety and tolerability.
Safety and Efficacy of Fenofibrate as a Treatment for Huntington's Disease.	Phase 2a, 6-month, randomized, double-blind, placebo-controlled study. **Active, not recruiting.**	NCT03515213	DM	Fenofibrate 145 mg.	20	This study will test the safety and effectiveness of fenofibrate to treat HD.
Nilotinib in Huntington's Disease (Tasigna HD).	Phase 1b; open-label, proof of concept study. **Recruiting**	NCT03764215	S/DM	Nilotinib 150 and 300 mg	10	Previous data on patients with Parkinson's disease and Dementia with Lewy Bodies were compelling to evaluate the effects of Nilotinib in an open label proof-of-concept study in patients with HD.
Within Subject Crossover Study of Cognitive Effects of Neflamapimod in Early-Stage Huntington Disease.	Phase 2; 10-week, randomized, double-blind, placebo-controlled crossover study. **Recruiting**	NCT03980938	DM	Neflamapimod 40 mg.	16	This study will test the ability of Neflamapimod to reverse hippocampal dysfunction in patients with early stage HD.

Table 2. (Continued)

Study Title	Phase/Design	Registration ID	S or DM	Intervention/ Treatment	N	Study Status/Results
Symptomatic treatment						
A Pilot Study Assessing Impulsivity in Patients With Huntington's Disease on Xenazine (Tetrabenazine).	Phase 4; open-label assessment of behavioral symptoms. **Recruiting.**	NCT02509793	S	Tetrabenazine.	20	This study will evaluate whether or not tetrabenazine reduces impulsivity in HD patients. Other behavioral symptoms including depression and suicidal ideations will also be evaluated.
Symptomatic Therapy for Patients With Huntington's Disease.	Phase 1; randomized, open-label, single group assignment study. **Recruiting**	NCT04071639		Haloperidol, Risperidone and Zoloft	100	The purpose of the study is to evaluate symptomatic treatment regimen efficacy based on different disease stages.
Efficacy and Safety of SOM3355 in Huntington's Disease Chorea.	Phase 2a; double-blind, placebo-controlled, multiple ascending dose study. **Active, not recruiting.**	NCT03575676	S	SOM3355 100 or 200 mg twice a day.	30	This study will evaluate the effectiveness of SOM3355 in treating chorea associated with HD.
Evaluating the Efficacy of Dextromethorphan/Quinidine in Treating Irritability in Huntington's Disease.	Phase 3; randomized, double-blind, placebo-controlled, crossover study. **Recruiting**	NCT03854019	S	Dextromethorphan/quinidine 20mg/10mg	22	This study will evaluate efficacy and safety of dextromethorphan/quinidine in reducing irritability in HD patients.
Non-pharmacological interventions						
Deep Brain Stimulation (DBS) of the Globus Pallidus (GP) in Huntington's Disease (HD) (HD-DBS).	Randomized, controlled, parallel assignment (stimulation vs. non-stimulation) study. **Recruiting.**	NCT02535884	S	ACTIVA® PC neurostimulator (Model 37601)	50	This study will test the safety and efficacy of pallidal DBS.

Study Title	Phase/Design	Registration ID	S or DM	Intervention/ Treatment	N	Study Status/Results
Non-pharmacological interventions						
ExAblate Transcranial MRgFUS for the Management of Treatment-Refractory Movement Disorders.	Open-label, single-group assignment study. **Recruiting**.	NCT02252380	S	Transcranial ExAblate System	10	The purpose of this study is to evaluate the safety and initial effectiveness of MRI-guided focused ultrasound thermal ablation of a designated area in the brain of patients suffering from movement disorder symptoms.
Brain Stimulation in Movement Disorders.	Randomized, double-blind, crossover study. **Unknown status.**	NCT02216474	DM	Transcranial direct current stimulation	100	This trial will explore the effects of very gentle electrical stimulation of the brain in patients with movement disorders.
Physical Activity and Exercise Outcomes in Huntington's Disease (PACE-HD).	Open-label, randomized, 12-month, a longitudinal cohort study. **Recruiting.**	NCT03344601	S	Physical exercise	120	This study evaluates the effects of physical exercise on HD patients (comparing a supported structured aerobic exercise training program to activity as usual).

Minocycline is a second-generation tetracycline that has been in therapeutic use for over 30 years. The evidence that minocycline exerts neuroprotective effects in rodent models of neurodegenerative diseases, including HD (Li, Yuan, and Schluesener 2013) motivated further investigation in clinical trials with patients with HD. A clinical study (NCT00277355) showed that minocycline at 100 and 200 mg/day was well tolerated during 8-week treatment with 60 patients with HD. However, no efficacy was observed, with no effect on the UHDRS or cognitive tests scores (Huntington Study Group 2004). The short time period treatment might explain the lack of efficacy. An 18-month protocol was then designed (NCT00277355), but here again minocycline 200 mg/day was considered safe and well tolerated with no noticeable changes were reported in cognitive and motor symptoms. The small decline in total functional capacity (TFC) score in the minocycline group suggested futility; and the evidence was considered insufficient to justify a larger and longer trial of minocycline in HD (D.I. Huntington Study Group 2010).

Recently, another study targeting the immune system in HD gene carriers emerged as a potential HD-modifying therapy. The SIGNAL trial is a phase 2, multi-center, randomized, double-blind, placebo-controlled study that assess the safety, tolerability, pharmacokinetics, and efficacy of Pepinemab VX15/2503 ("VX15") in subjects with late prodromal and early manifest HD (NCT02481674). VX15/2503 is an antibody to semaphorin 4D (SEM4D) that regulates the activation and migration of inflammatory cells and inhibits the differentiation of oligodendrocyte precursors in the brain. The inhibition of SEM4D signaling could decrease central nervous system (CNS) inflammation, increase neuronal outgrowth and enhance oligodendrocyte maturation, which may be of therapeutic benefit in the treatment of HD (E.S. Smith et al. 2015). This trial was based on promising pre-clinical data. In the YAC128 transgenic HD mouse model, the anti-SEM4D treatment improved neuropathological signatures, including striatal, cortical, and corpus callosum atrophy and prevented testicular degeneration. In parallel, behavioral symptoms were also improved, including reduction in the anxiety-like behavior and rescue of cognitive deficits (Southwell et al. 2015). The estimated date for the Signal study final data collection of the primary outcome measure is May 2020. The first 36 participants have completed six months of study intervention, but detailed results have not been released.

Metabolic- and Mitochondrial-Based Protective Strategies

Therapeutic strategies targeting antioxidant and metabolic pathways have also been tested in the HD population. A clinical trial called 2CARE (NCT00608881) was designed several years ago to test the hypothesis that the chronic treatment of patients in early-stage HD with high-dosage coenzyme Q10 (CoQ10) would slow the functional decline over a 60-month follow-up. CoQ plays a central role in oxidative phosphorylation, appears to stabilize membranes, acts as an antioxidant (Pepping 1999) and may influence vesicle migration, cell growth, and signal transmission (Musumeci et al. 2001). The 2CARE study randomly assigned 609 subjects with early-HD to 2,400 mg/day of CoQ10 or placebo and planned to follow subjects for 5 years. At the time of study termination, only 34% of the 609 enrolled patients had completed the month 60 visit (25% on study drug and 9% off study drug), and 42% were still active in the trial (34% on study drug and 8% off study drug). In addition, 18% of participants had withdrawn participation in the trial while alive (12% on study drug and 6% off study drug at time of withdrawal), and 5.7% died during study participation (3.0% on study drug and 2.8% off study drug). CoQ10 was generally safe and well-tolerated. However, no statistically significant differences were observed between treatment groups (i.e., CoQ10 *vs.* placebo) for the primary or secondary outcome measures. A futility analysis failed to show likelihood of benefit of CoQ10 in HD and the trial was then terminated (McGarry, McDermott, et al. 2017).

Two other clinical trials were designed to evaluate safety and efficacy of CoQ10 treatment in HD. The PREQUEL study (NCT00920699) sought to assess the change from baseline to 20 weeks on biomarkers of oxidative stress [8-Hydroxydeoxyguanosine (8OHdG) and 8-Hydroxyguanosine (8OHrG)] and DNA repair mechanisms [8-Oxoguanine DNA Glycosylase

(OGG1)] in pre-manifest HD participants treated with CoQ10. The trial was completed and again CoQ10 was generally safe and well tolerated . CoQ10 treatment was associated with increases in serum levels of CoQ10, but with no change in 8OHdG levels. Also, there was no relationship between 8OHdG level and predicted age of disease onset (C. Ross, Biglan, et al. 2014; Biglan et al. 2014). Lastly, the purpose of NCT00980694 study was to determine if people that switch from the common formulation of CoQ10 ("ubiquinone") to a different formulation ("ubiquinol") have higher levels of CoQ10 in their blood after taking the same dose. The study has been completed but no results were published up to date. Taken together, the data do not justify use of CoQ10 as a treatment to slow functional decline in HD

Another therapeutic strategy tested the efficacy of creatine for HD. Creatine is a nutritional supplement that is converted to phosphocreatine, which acts as a high-energy phosphate source for restoring adenosine triphosphate (ATP) from adenosine diphosphate (Andres, Wallimann, and Widmer 2016). In pre-clinical studies with transgenic mouse models of HD, creatine was able to delay the onset and slow the progression of behavioral and pathologic HD phenotypes. In addition, it reversed cerebral ATP deficiency and extended survival in a dose-dependent manner (Dedeoglu et al. 2003). Initially, three double-blind placebo-controlled clinical trials of creatine were performed, but two clinical trials found no difference between placebo and treatment groups in regards to functional and cognitive status (S.M. Hersch et al. 2006; Verbessem et al. 2003). Although clinical measures were unchanged over the treatment course, the CREST-HD study (NCT00026988) showed that creatine 8g/day resulted in an increase in serum and brain creatine concentrations, which returned to baseline after washout. Serum 8OHdG levels, an indicator of oxidative injury to DNA, were markedly elevated in HD and reduced by creatine treatment (S.M. Hersch et al. 2006)

Another trial, called PRECREST (NCT00592995) enrolled 64 people with premanifest HD, who were randomly allocated to 15 g of creatinine twice daily (30 g per day) or placebo for a 6-month double-blind phase, followed by a 12-month open-label extension (PRECREST-X, NCT01411150). There was a treatment-dependent slowing of cortical and striatal atrophy, but no improvement in memory or cognitive tests (Rosas et al. 2014). Open-label extension studies [CREST-X (NCT01412151) and PRECREST-2X (NCT01411163)] were then designed to further assess the long-term safety and tolerability of creatine treatment in HD. The studies have been completed but there are no results available. Another study, called CREST-E (NCT00712426) was designed to further investigate these contradictory results. The CREST-E study randomly assigned 553 subjects to up to 40 g of creatine or placebo and planned to follow subjects for 3 years. The trial was terminated early because preliminary analysis revealed that the futility stopping criterion had been reached, indicating a high possibility that the study, if completed, would not exhibit a positive effect of creatine. No safety concerns were noted. Taken together, the data do not support the use of creatine treatment for delaying functional decline in early-manifest HD (S.M. Hersch et al. 2017).

Phosphodiesterase 10A (PDE10A) is a substrate enzyme highly expressed in the striatal medium spiny neurons. PDE10A regulates cyclic adenosine monophosphate (cAMP) and cyclic guanosine monophosphate (cGMP) downstream signaling cascades. It has been hypothesized that the toxic effects of mHTT on PDE10A are detrimental for neuronal survival and for the regulation of basal ganglia functions. Therefore, Pfizer launched a study to assess safety, tolerability, and efficacy of a PDE10A inhibitor (PF-02545920) in patients with HD. The first trial (NCT01806896) showed that the experimental drug was generally safe tolerated. In addition, patients receiving PF-02545920 showed a significant improvement in their physical effort in response to incentive motivation during a grip-strength test. The Amaryllis clinical trial (NCT02197130) was then designed to assess safety, tolerability and the efficacy of a 26-week treatment with PF-0254592 on motor function in HD patients, as well as obtain safety and exploratory efficacy data in a 12-month open-label extension study (NCT02342548). At the end of the 26-week, double-blind, placebo-controlled, randomized trial, there was no evidence of efficacy in primary (change in UHDRS-TMS score) or secondary clinical endpoints with PF02545920 5 mg or 20 mg twice a day (M. Delnomdedieu et al. 2018).Based on these results, decision was made to terminate the open-label extension study and the overall PDE10 HD program was terminated (M. Delnomdedieu 2018).

Mitochondrial dysfunction is regarded as one of the mechanisms contributing to neurodegeneration in HD. Oxidative stress may mediate the final pathway of neuronal loss and result in membrane instability. Therefore, the effects of ethyl-eicosapentaenoic acid (ethyl-EPA) in HD have been tested. The investigators hypothesized that this ω-3 fatty acid could be beneficial for HD by stabilizing membranes and inhibiting apoptosis. The TREND-HD trial (NCT00146211) was a phase 3, 6-month, randomized, double-blind, placebo-controlled study with 316 patients with mild to moderate HD. The results were disappointing: the ethyl-EPA treatment resulted in no beneficial effects in measures of motor function, global functioning cognition, or global impression (Huntington Study Group 2008). The TRIHEP2 trial (NCT01882062) showed that 1-month treatment with another fatty acid, triheptanoin, was able to correct the brain bioenergetic profile (based on the inorganic phosphate /phosphocreatine ratio) in early stage HD (Adanyeguh et al. 2015). The TRIHEP3 trial (NCT02453061) is currently ongoing and it will evaluate the effect of triheptanoin oil on brain energy restoration and caudate atrophy in 100 patients with HD. Secondary outcomes include motor, cognitive, behavior and functionality measures, in addition to safety and tolerability.

Another experimental drug called latrepirdine (dimebon) was the interest of a group of trials based on mitochondrial dysfunction impairment in HD. Latrepirdine was initially developed as an antihistamine and subsequently was shown to stabilize mitochondrial membranes and function. The first trial (NCT00387270) was planned to assess safety study (phase 1/2) in 9 patients with HD receiving 10 or 20 mg of latrepirdine 3 times a day. The trial has been completed but no results have been published. In a randomized trial of latrepirdine in 91 individuals with mild to moderate HD, latrepirdine was found to be safe and well tolerated during 3 months of treatment (NCT00387270). In addition, compared with placebo, latrepirdine treatment resulted in a discrete but significant improvement in one of the cognitive scales (mini-mental state examination, MMSE), but not with improvement in other cognitive outcome measures (Kieburtz et al. 2010).

Based on the results of this phase 2 study, the HORIZON study was planned (NCT00920946). This was a multicenter, 26-week, randomized, double-blind, placebo-controlled study of latrepirdine to assess its efficacy in improving cognition and global function in patients with mild to moderate HD. Here again, latrepirdine was safe and well tolerated. However, the treatment did not improve cognition or global function in patients with HD with baseline cognitive impairment (Horizon Investigators of the Huntington Study Group and European Huntington's Disease Network 2013). The open-label extension of the HORIZON protocol (HORIZON PLUS, NCT01085266) was terminated because of the unsuccessful HORIZON trial results.

Other Disease-Modifying Therapies

Studies with HD mouse models have shown an involvement of the endocannabinoid system in the pathogenesis of HD. Because of this, a double-blind, randomized, placebo-controlled, cross-over pilot clinical trial has been conducted to assess safety, tolerability, and efficacy of Sativex® in patients with HD (NCT01502046). Sativex® is a botanical extract with an equimolecular combination of delta-9-tetrahydrocannabinol and cannabidiol. Safety and tolerability were confirmed but no differences on motor, cognitive, behavioral and functional scores were detected as compared to placebo (Lopez-Sendon Moreno et al. 2016).

Other strategies, such as antiglutamatergic drugs have been tried as potential disease-modifying therapies for HD and will be discussed in the next section.

PHARMACOLOGICAL TREATMENT FOR HD SYMPTOMS

Despite significant efforts to find an effective disease-modifying therapy, pharmacological interventions to stop or delay the process underlying HD pathophysiology are not yet available. While a great deal is known about the *HTT* gene, the pathogenesis of HD is not fully understood and several mechanisms might be involved. The treatment of HD is currently focused on improving daily functioning and quality of life by reducing symptoms' burden (Coppen and Roos 2017). Remarkable progress is being made in HD symptomatic treatment, but we are still far from the ideal scenario. Currently, there are two FDA-approved medications for the treatment of chorea in HD: the type 2 vesicular monoamine transporter (VMAT2) inhibitor tetrabenazine (TBZ) and its deuterated form with an improved pharmacokinetic profile, deutetrabenzine. Antipsychotics such as haloperidol and risperidone have also been traditionally used to treat chorea, but these drugs may result in a variety of adverse effects, including Parkinsonism and tardive dyskinesia (Testa and Jankovic 2019). The NEUROHD (NCT00632645) was a 12-month, randomized, open-label study compared beneficial and adverse effects of olanzapine, tiapride, and tetrabenazine in patients with HD. This trial was completed in 2018, however, no results have been published to date. It is worth mentioning that despite thecommon use of antipsychotics to treat HD chorea, a Cochrane review concluded that TBZ is the antichoreic medication with best available clinical evidence. This review was published in 2009 when deutetrabenazine was not yet available (T. Mestre et al. 2009). The use of antipsychotics persists in many regions, in part due to the enormous differences in cost between VMAT2 inhibitors and antipsychotics (Testa and Jankovic 2019).

Regarding the non-motor symptoms in HD, although there are several strategies and pharmacological options available, there is currently insufficient data for evidence-based guidelines on the management of these common symptoms. In the absence of strong clinical data, expert opinion-based recommendations may provide practical guidance (Testa and Jankovic 2019). Clinical experience has shown that most of the HD-related neuropsychiatric symptoms are treatable using pharmacologic and nonpharmacologic strategies developed for use in other populations. However, most of these strategies have not been specifically tested in the HD population. The management of cognitive and psychiatric symptoms in HD can be complex because several conditions often co-exist and differ according to disease stage. The treatment should be optimized to cover different symptoms while limiting polypharmacy (Anderson et al. 2018). In this regard, we highlight the relevance of clinical trials to assess the efficacy of drugs to treat motor and non-motor symptoms in HD population at different stages. Among the vast repertoire of medications used to treat non-motor symptoms in HD, only some of them have been tested in registered clinical trials.

Atomoxetine (Strattera) is a nonstimulant norepinephrine reuptake inhibitor used to treat attention deficit hyperactivity disorder (ADHD). Because atomoxetine has successfully improved attention and executive functions in children and adults with ADHD, it has been hypothesized that this drug would be effective in HD-related cognitive impairments. A 10-week, randomized, double-blind, placebo-controlled, crossover study (NCT00368849) demonstrated no advantages of atomoxetine over placebo in attention, psychiatric, and motor symptom scores in patients with early HD (Beglinger et al. 2009). Another trial was conducted to assess the effectiveness of citalopram in improve executive function in HD (NCT00271596). Citalopram is a selective serotonin reuptake inhibitor widely used in clinical practice for the treatment of depressive disorders, with proved cognitive-enhancing properties. However, the randomized, placebo-controlled pilot study (NCT00271596) failed to show that short-term (20 weeks) treatment with citalopram improved executive functions in patients with HD with cognitive complaints. Of note, citalopram improved mood in non-depressed patients (patients with active depression were not included in the study), thus raising the possibility of efficacy for subsyndromal depression in HD (Beglinger et al. 2014).

A clinical trial with another antidepressant, bupropion, has been conducted as an attempt to treat apathy in HD. Apathy is one of the most common non-motor symptoms in HD, correlating directly with disease progression. Bupropion is a norepinephrine/dopamine reuptake inhibitor, thereby potentially increasing DA neurotransmission in areas relevant for apathy. Although single case-reports and results of small series suggested the effectiveness of bupropion for the treatment of apathy in HD and other neurodegenerative diseases, the results of Action-HD (NCT01914965) were disappointing. In this 10-week, randomized, double-blind, placebo-controlled, crossover study bupropion did not alleviate apathy in HD. Interestingly, study participation improved symptoms of apathy, regardless of whether the drug or the placebo was administered (Gelderblom et al. 2017).

Type 2 Vesicular Monoamine Transporter (VMAT2) Inhibitors

TBZ (Xenazine) and Deutetrabenazine (Austedo) are currently the only two medications approved by the FDA specifically to treat chorea in individuals with HD.

TBZ is a VMAT-2 inhibitor thus leading to depletion of monoamines, particularly dopamine in the brain (Yero and Rey 2008). The effective and safe use of TBZ to treat chorea was first reported in 1988 by Jankovic and Orman (Jankovic and Orman 1988). Almost two decades later, a randomized clinical trial assessing the efficacy and safety of TBZ in HD chorea (NCT00219804) was performed. TBZ significantly reduced chorea burden, improved global outcome, and was generally safe and well tolerated in the 12-week double-blind study (Huntington Study Group 2006). In the open-label extension study, TBZ continued to effectively suppress chorea for up to 80 weeks and was generally well tolerated (Frank 2009). The effectiveness of TBZ in reducing chorea was further corroborated by a study showing the reemergence of chorea after TBZ treatment withdrawal (Frank et al. 2008). TBZ effects have been demonstrated to be beyond the improvement of chorea. TBZ withdrawal also resulted in decreased cognitive performance, as demonstrated by a significant deterioration in Stroop color-word scores in a clinical trial with 10 patients (NCT01834911) (Fekete, Davidson, and Jankovic 2012). TBZ use also improved balance and functional mobility in individuals with HD (NCT01451463) (Kegelmeyer et al. 2014). In addition, the risk of developing a metabolic syndrome or tardive dyskinesia is lower with TBZ than seen in antipsychotic drugs (Coppen and Roos 2017).

Despite recognized safety, tolerability, and efficacy for the treatment of HD chorea, TBZ use is associated with adverse symptoms that can limit its use, such as sedation, insomnia, fatigue, akathisia, anxiety, depression and suicidal behavior. These effects are related to peak concentrations of TBZ. In addition, TBZ is subject to variable CYP2D6 metabolism and often requires 3-times-a-day dosing. Therefore, new trials were conducted with deutetrabenazine, an isotopic isomer of TBZ with an improved pharmacokinetic profile. In deutetrabenazine, 6 deuterium atoms replace 6 hydrogen atoms in key positions, strengthening the carbon-deuterium compared to carbon-hydrogen bonds. As a result, deutetrabenazine is a molecule with longer half-life (requiring less frequent and lower daily doses) and reduced metabolic variability compared to TBZ, without changing target pharmacology. The lower peak concentrations and simplified dosing results in an improved risk-benefit profile of the modified version of TBZ (Huntington Study Group et al. 2016). The results of the two placebo-controlled, randomized clinical trials with deutetrabenazine were positive. Deutetrabenazine treatment significantly improved chorea control together with improvements in patient-centered end-points in comparison with placebo (NCT01795859) (Huntington Study Group et al. 2016). In addition, safety and tolerability of deutetrabenazine was comparable to that of TBZ and the overnight conversion to deutetrabenazine therapy provided a favorable safety profile and effectively maintained chorea control (NCT01897896) (Frank et al. 2017).

TBZ and deutetrabenazine will most likely define HD chorea treatment for years to come. Deutetrabenazine seems to have advantages over TBZ, because of the potential improved tolerance and adherence. However, the two drugs have yet to be tested in a true head-to-head study, so a concrete resolution has yet to be solidified. A host of clinical trials comparing the two drugs is required to reach the better conclusions (Dean and Sung 2018).

Dopaminergic Stabilizers

Pridopidine (ACR16) is as a competitive, low-affinity dopamine D2 antagonist with fast-off receptor-dissociation kinetics and with a slight preference for the agonist binding site (Waters et al. 2018). Pridopidine is dopidine, a pharmacological class of dopaminergic stabilizers. Pridopidine modulates hyperactivity or hypoactivity of the dopaminergic system, without having major effects on normal psychomotor function (Coppen and Roos 2017). Preclinical studies using different animal models of HD (R/6 and YAC128mice) have demonstrated that pridopidine can ameliorate HD-like behavior and be neuroprotective (Squitieri et al. 2015; Garcia-Miralles et al. 2017; Kusko et al. 2018). Unfortunately, clinical trials results were not as encouraging as the preclinical evidence. Pridopidine was safe and well tolerated but failed to achieve its primary efficacy outcomes (modified motor score) in two trials [MermaiHD (NCT00665223) and HART (NCT00724048)] (de Yebenes et al. 2011; H.I. Huntington Study Group 2013). The consistent effects on secondary outcomes related to motor abilities motivated the development of more trials in this regard. Open-HART (NCT01306929) and PRIDE-HD (NCT02006472) were then conducted but they failed to show any effectiveness of pridopidine in improving motor score or altering disease progression (McGarry, Kieburtz, et al. 2017; R. Reilmann et al. 2019). The open-label extension of the PRIDE study (Open-PRIDE, NCT02494778) was terminated.

Antiglutamatergic Drugs

mHTT elicits multiple cellular dysfunctions including an increase of glutamate-mediated excitotoxicity. Accordingly, targeting the excess of glutamate has been the goal for promising drugs leading to clinical trials in HD (Anglada-Huguet et al. 2017). In this regard, amantadine, memantine, mavoglurant, and riluzole and have been tested in HD.

Amantadine and memantine are N-methyl-D-aspartic acid (NMDA) receptor antagonists. Amantadine is commonly used in the treatment of levodopa-induced dyskinesias in Parkinson's disease and memantine is used in moderate to severe Alzheimer's disease. Amantadine has been recommended as an alternative for TBZ by the 2012 American Academy of Neurology (AAN) guidelines for the pharmacological treatment of HD chorea (Armstrong, Miyasaki, and American Academy of Neurology 2012).

The treatment with amantadine resulted in significant improvement of motor symptoms in two different trials with patients with HD. In a 2-week, randomized, double-blind, placebo-controlled, crossover trial, amantadine 400 mg daily reduced UHDRS chorea extremity score at rest in 36% (Verhagen Metman et al. 2002). In addition, an open-label study showed that a one-year treatment with amantadine 100 mg daily resulted in a 9-point reduction in the UHDRS score (Lucetti et al. 2002). However, the only clinical trial registered at ClinicalTrials.gov (NCT00001930) failed to prove amantadine effectiveness in the treatment of HD chorea. In this 2-week, randomized, placebo-controlled, crossover trial, amantadine was not effective for HD chorea, although most patients felt subjectively better during the amantadine treatment (O'Suilleabhain and Dewey 2003). The MITIGATE-HD is a 24-week, randomized, double-blind, placebo-controlled study has been registered in 2011 (NCT014584700) aiming at assessing the safety and effectiveness of memantine in treating neuropsychiatric and cognitive symptoms in early-HD. Although the trial has been completed in 2014, no results have been published.

Mavoglurant (AFQ056) is a metabotropic glutamate receptor 5 (mGluR5) antagonist. This experimental drug has shown antidyskinetic properties in clinical trials with patients with Parkinson's disease with levodopa-induced dyskinesia (Berg et al. 2011; Stocchi et al. 2013), leading to the hypothesis that this drug would be effective for chorea in HD. However, a 32-day randomized, double-blind, placebo-controlled study with mavoglurant (NCT01019473) was terminated because no improvement was observed on the primary outcomes. The drug was was well tolerated but did not reduce chorea in HD (R. Reilmann et al. 2015).

Riluzole modulates glutamate neurotransmission by inhibiting both glutamate release and postsynatpic glutamate receptor signaling. To date, riluzole is the only FDA-approved drug to treat amyotrophic lateral sclerosis. Although the riluzole treatment has been neuroprotective, reducing the progression of neurological abnormalities in the R/6 mice model of HD (Schiefer et al. 2002), a 3-year, randomized, double-blind, placebo-controlled study (NCT00277602) failed to demonstrate any neuroprotective or beneficial symptomatic effects of riluzole in a cohort of

537 patients with HD (379 completed the study) (Landwehrmeyer et al. 2007).

NON-PHARMACOLOGICAL TRIALS IN HD

Cognitive and Other Mental Health Therapies

Cognitive therapy is a non-invasive form of treatment in patients with HD. It is not describedto be a disease-modifying treatment; however, it may offertemporary symptomatic improvement. "Brain exercises" can put some control back in the patients' hands. Becuase HD is a progressive disease for which there is not yet a cure, patients often feel as if they have lost control of their own life. The relatively simple methods that have been tested demonstrated positive results.Cognitive therapy can greatly improve a patient's mental health by improving both memory and mental well-being. In a disease for which common symptoms include apathy and suicidal thoughts, mental well-being is crucial to maintain. Various clinical trials have assessed the viability of cognitive therapy using computerized cognitive training programs, music, and even laughter therapy.

Computerized training programs such as Lumosity have been widely proven to improve cognitive capacity and abilities in the general population. A study completed in March 2016 tested the ability of a memory-training program called CogMed QM to improve nine prodromal HD and early manifest patients' memory (NCT02926820). Scores on the neuropsychological assessments digit span, spatial span, symbol span, and auditory working memory were compared before and after the 25-session (5 weeks) training program. All patients that adhered to the program reported seeing improvement and showed significant improvement in the neuropsychological assessments. This study concluded that the memory training software CogMed QM could be beneficial for patients' working memory, but a large-scale intervention would need to be done to further investigate (Sadeghi et al. 2017).

Another study completed in March 2019 explored a related but slightly different cognitive training program called CogTrainHD (NCT02990676). 30 manifest HD patients were asked to complete 30 minutes of training 3 days a week for 12 weeks. Motor and cognitive assessments were conducted at the start and end of the study to determine the effect the training had on patients' abilities in those two areas (Yhnell et al. 2018).. Results have not yet been published.

An additional form of non-pharmacological therapy tested in HD patients is music therapy, which uses music to improve everything from communication skills to physical rehabilitation and facilitating movement. In addition, music therapy can increase patients' motivation to continue treatment as well as provide an emotional outlet for patients to express their feelings (American Music Therapy Association). A phase 1 clinical trial completed in June 2010 gave patients one 30-minute individual music therapy session every other week and one 1-hour group music therapy each month, for a period of three months, measuring their UHDRS score before and after the study (NCT00178360). Four out of the 5 patients reported positive feelings towards the program, and the UHDRS scores improved for finger tapping, pronation/supination and the Luria. However, the sample size was too small to reach statistical significance, therefore, alarger study must be done to accurately determine the potential positive effects of music therapy.

Another nonpharamaclogic treatment option is laughter therapy, which has been used to treat illnesses by "strengthening breathing muscles, improving mood, and providing pain and stress relief." This study, completed in August 2018 tested the efficacy of laughter therapy in treating mood, stress, and self-efficacy problems in patients with CNS disorders (NCT02750982). The study will measure the effect of laughter therapy on patients' scores on various tests: PHQ-9 (a depression patient questionnaire), GAD-7 (for generalized anxiety disorder), and the GSE (general self-efficacy scale). Results are pending.

Physical Therapy

Physical therapy has a wide range of applications, but it is most commonly used to strengthen an area of weakness after an injury and/or surgery or slow the decline of motor strength and flexibility associated with old age and/or degenerative disease. Both of these applications improve strength and mobility in the short run, but differ in their long-term goals. Unlike post-injury/surgical rehabilitation, the physical therapy used in patients with neurodegenerative diseases like HD improve symptomsSimilar to cognitive therapy, physical therapy can provide patients with the all-important control over their own lives that is seemingly taken away with a diagnosis of HD. Several clinical trials have been done to assess the effect of physical therapy on patients with HD, most of which generally have similar results: exercise training seems to be safe and feasible in HD patients, holding the potential to improve motor symptoms and quality of life I individuals with HD.

Video games have long been advertised to have negative effects on those who play them, purportedly affecting everything from relationships with friends and family to increased aggression and even depression. However, the benefits of playing video games have been also recognized and a more balanced perspective is needed (Granic, Lobel, and Engels 2014). In this regard, a study was completed in June 2012 to test the possible positive effects of a certain video game (*Dance, Dance, Revolution*) on balance, gait, and mobility. This therapist-guided Video-game Biofeedback Modulated Exercise (ViBE) program also aimed to improve fall risk, neuropsychological symptoms, and overall quality of life (NCT01735981). Most participants enjoyed the program and saw improvements in movement; *Dance, Dance, Revolution* had a positive impact on HD patients and is a safe method of exercise intervention (Kloos et al. 2013).

A study completed in September 2016 tested whether treadmill-walking sessions could lead to improved gait in patients with Lewy Body dementia and HD (NCT02268617). No results have been published to date. Studies with the CAG_{140} knock-in mouse model of HD indicate that treadmill exercise ameliorated HD-like behaviors and exerted neuroprotective effects (Stefanko et al. 2017).

A trial completed in July 2016 used kinesthetic tests and psychological questionnaires to test the possible positive effect that contemporary dance practice has, not only on movement associated with HD but also on emotions and empathy. In addition, it evaluated how patients' partners and caregivers described the patients' movements and how they changed over the course of the practice plan (NCT01842919). Results showed widespread motor improvement over the course of the 5 months, with patients reporting that it greatly altered the way they "felt and lived in their bodies" (Trinkler et al. 2019).

In a trial completed in January 2018 (NCT01879267), researchers tested whether endurance exercise could stabilize or even reverse the "PGC-1a dependent alterations of muscle function and structure" seen in HD patients. Using a 6-month endurance training program, 20 male participants with HD were tested against 20 healthy males completing the same program. The aim of this study was to assess the difference in metabolic and physiological improvement in each group. Both groups showed improvement, and the mitochondria of skeletal muscle in HD patients were equally responsive to exercise program as those in the healthy controls (Mueller et al. 2017).

A trial completed in April 2019 tested the feasibility and acceptability of physical activity coaching in patients with pre-manifest and early stage HD (NCT03306888). No trial to date had tested the effect of these patient types, which may stand to gain the most from exercise. The results have yet to be posted from this trial.

Another, larger study currently recruiting will explicitly test the relationship between physical activity and disease progression by assessing VO2 max using wearable activity monitors. In addition, it will test the feasibility of sustained exercise (longer than 3 months) in HD patients. The goal is to provide the necessary information for exercise to be able to be used as a therapeutic intervention for HD (NCT03344601). The results will hopefully give insight into the process of using exercise therapeutically in HD.

Scheduled to be completed in 2021, a study is currently underway examining the multitasking habits of people with neurological disease. Specifically, researchers are examining the difference in patients' walking while performing a cognitive task (talking) simultaneously and when walking alone. The goal of the study is to assess the effectiveness of a combination of cognitive training and treadmill walking against one of the two alone. Results have yet to be posted since the study has not been completed.

CONCLUSION

Despite significant advances in our understanding of HD, a disease-modifying therapy remains elusive. While a great deal is known about the HTT gene, the pathogenesis is not fully understood. Based on data from preclinical studies, clinical trials have been conducted targeting different aspects of HD pathology, such as mHTT aggregation, neurodegeneration, immune/inflammatory mechanisms, glutamate-mediated excitotoxicity, the dopaminergic pathway, and mitochondrial dysfunction. None of these trials has been successful in identifying a drug with proven efficacy to modify HD progression, and thus for the moment, these agents have no role to play in the standard care of patients with HD. Several factors might influence the disappointing results, including underpowered studies and the lack of sufficient clinical and biological markers capable of tracking disease modification. The clinical scales currently used as primary endpoints might not be sensitive in detecting signs and symptoms of disease progression. New innovative tools to objectively assess disease signs and symptoms, and the development of neuroimaging- or biological fluid-based markers of disease progression will be imperative to the success of clinical trials in HD. The recent advances in therapeutic strategies promise an exciting era for clinical trials in HD. Current and future trials are focusing on lowering the mHTT, by targeting mHTT production, aggregation, misfolding, and removal.

While HD is not curable, symptomatic treatments are available aimed at improving patients' quality of life and functionality. Clinical experience indicates that most of the HD-related symptoms are treatable using pharmacologic and non-pharmacologic strategies. The pharmacologic management of HD is complex because of the coexistence of motor and nonmotor symptoms, therefore treatment decisions should be adapted to address all symptoms while limiting polypharmacy. Currently, many of the proposed treatments are based on expert opinions. Randomized controlled trials are needed to study the best treatment options for the various symptoms associated with HD. HD is a multifaceted disease and therefore requires a multifaceted treatment approach Attention should paid to the importance of interdisciplinary, comprehensive care including cognitive-behavioral therapy, physical, occupational and speech therapy and nutritional services, social work and genetic counseling services. Increased recognition of the phenotypic variability in HD can also improve the symptomatic treatment goals. It is imperative that care providers acknowledge the complexities of the disease for both the patient and the family providing nonpharmacologic and pharmacologic treatment throughout the disease course.

REFERENCES

Adanyeguh, I. M., Rinaldi, D., Henry, P. G., Caillet, S., Valabregue, R., Durr, A. & Mochel, F. (2015). "Triheptanoin improves brain energy metabolism in patients with Huntington disease." *Neurology, 84* (5), 490-5. https://doi.org/10.1212/WNL.0000000000001214. https://www.ncbi.nlm.nih.gov/pubmed/25568297.

American Music Therapy Association. *What is Music Therapy.* https://www.musictherapy.org/about/musictherapy.

Anderson, K. E., van Duijn, E., Craufurd, D., Drazinic, C., Edmondson, M., Goodman, N., van Kammen, D., Loy, C., Priller, J. & Goodman, L. V. (2018). "Clinical Management of Neuropsychiatric Symptoms of Huntington Disease: Expert-Based Consensus Guidelines on Agitation,

Anxiety, Apathy, Psychosis and Sleep Disorders." *J Huntingtons Dis*, 7 (3), 355-366. https://doi.org/10.3233/JHD-180293. https:// www.ncbi. nlm.nih.gov/pubmed/30040737.

Andres, R. H., Wallimann, T. & Widmer, H. R. (2016). "Creatine supplementation improves neural progenitor cell survival in Huntington's disease." *Brain Circ*, 2 (3), 133-137. https://doi.org/ 10.4103/2394-8108.192519. https://www.ncbi.nlm.nih.gov/ pubmed/ 30276289.

Anglada-Huguet, M., Vidal-Sancho, L., Cabezas-Llobet, N., Alberch, J. & Xifró, X (2017). "Pathogenesis of Huntington's Disease: How to Fight Excitotoxicity and Transcriptional Dysregulation." In *Huntington's Disease - Molecular Pathogenesis and Current Models*, edited by N.E. Tunalı, 37-73. Croatia: InTech.

Armstrong, M. J., Miyasaki, J. M. & American Academy of Neurology. (2012). "Evidence-based guideline: pharmacologic treatment of chorea in Huntington disease: report of the guideline development subcommittee of the American Academy of Neurology." *Neurology*, 79 (6), 597-603. https://doi.org/10.1212/WNL.0b013e318263c443. https:// www.ncbi.nlm.nih.gov/pubmed/22815556.

Bachoud-Levi, A. C. (2017). "From open to large-scale randomized cell transplantation trials in Huntington's disease: Lessons from the multicentric intracerebral grafting in Huntington's disease trial (MIG-HD) and previous pilot studies." *Prog Brain Res*, 230, 227-261. https://doi.org/10.1016/bs.pbr.2016.12.011. https:// www.ncbi.nlm.nih. gov/pubmed/28552231.

Beglinger, L. J., Adams, W. H., Langbehn, D., Fiedorowicz, J. G., Jorge, R., Biglan, K., Caviness, J., Olson, B., Robinson, R. G., Kieburtz, K. & Paulsen, J. S. (2014). "Results of the citalopram to enhance cognition in Huntington disease trial." *Mov Disord*, 29 (3), 401-5. https:// doi.org/10.1002/mds.25750. https://www.ncbi.nlm.nih.gov/pubmed/24375941.

Beglinger, L. J., Adams, W. H., Paulson, H., Fiedorowicz, J. G., Langbehn, D. R., Duff, K., Leserman, A. & Paulsen, J. S. (2009). "Randomized controlled trial of atomoxetine for cognitive dysfunction in early

Huntington disease." *J Clin Psychopharmacol*, *29* (5), 484-7. https://doi.org/10.1097/JCP.0b013e3181b2ac0a. https:// www.ncbi.nlm.nih.gov/pubmed/19745649.

Berg, D., Godau, J., Trenkwalder, C., Eggert, K., Csoti, I., Storch, A., Huber, H., Morelli-Canelo, M., Stamelou, M., Ries, V., Wolz, M., Schneider, C., Di Paolo, T., Gasparini, F., Hariry, S., Vandemeulebroecke, M., Abi-Saab, W., Cooke, K., Johns, D. & Gomez-Mancilla, B. (2011). "AFQ056 treatment of levodopa-induced dyskinesias: results of 2 randomized controlled trials." *Mov Disord*, *26* (7), 1243-50. https://doi.org/10.1002/mds.23616. https://www.ncbi.nlm.nih.gov/ pub med/21484867.

Biglan, K., Ross, C., Killoran, A., Beal, M. F., Matson, W., Julian-Baros, E., Yoritomo, N., Gao, S., McDermott, M. & Huntington Study Group PREQUEL Investigators. (2014). "8OHdG Levels in Response to Coenzyme Q10 in the PREQUEL Study of Pre-manifest Huntington Disease." *Neurotherapeutics*, *11*, 223-224.

Biotech, Active, (2019). *The Phase 2 LEGATO-HD study of laquinimod in Huntington's disease.*

Cherny, R. A., Ayton, S., Finkelstein, D. I., Bush, A. I., McColl, G. & Massa, S. M. (2012). "PBT2 Reduces Toxicity in a C. elegans Model of polyQ Aggregation and Extends Lifespan, Reduces Striatal Atrophy and Improves Motor Performance in the R6/2 Mouse Model of Huntington's Disease." *J Huntingtons Dis*, *1* (2), 211-9. https:// doi.org/10.3233/JHD-120029. https://www.ncbi.nlm.nih.gov/pubmed/ 25063332.

Comi, G., Jeffery, D., Kappos, L., Montalban, X., Boyko, A., Rocca, M. A., Filippi, M. & Allegro Study Group. (2012). "Placebo-controlled trial of oral laquinimod for multiple sclerosis." *N Engl J Med*, *366* (11), 1000-9. https://doi.org/10.1056/NEJMoa1104318. https:// www.ncbi.nlm.nih.gov/pubmed/22417253.

Coppen, E. M. & Roos, R. A. (2017). "Current Pharmacological Approaches to Reduce Chorea in Huntington's Disease." *Drugs*, *77* (1), 29-46. https://doi.org/10.1007/s40265-016-0670-4. https:// www.ncbi.nlm.nih.gov/pubmed/27988871.

de Yebenes, J. G., Landwehrmeyer, B., Squitieri, F., Reilmann, R., Rosser, A., Barker, R. A., Saft, C., Magnet, M. K., Sword, A., Rembratt, A., Tedroff, J. & H. D. study investigators Mermai. (2011). "Pridopidine for the treatment of motor function in patients with Huntington's disease (MermaiHD): a phase 3, randomised, double-blind, placebo-controlled trial." *Lancet Neurol, 10* (12), 1049-57. https://doi.org/ 10.1016/S1474-4422(11)70233-2. https://www.ncbi.nlm.nih.gov/ pubmed/22071279.

Dean, M. & Sung, V. W. (2018). "Review of deutetrabenazine: a novel treatment for chorea associated with Huntington's disease." *Drug Des Devel Ther, 12,* 313-319. https://doi.org/10.2147/DDDT.S138828. https://www.ncbi.nlm.nih.gov/pubmed/29497277.

Dedeoglu, A., Kubilus, J. K., Yang, L., Ferrante, K. L., Hersch, S. M., Beal, M. F. & Ferrante, R. J. (2003). "Creatine therapy provides neuroprotection after onset of clinical symptoms in Huntington's disease transgenic mice." *J Neurochem, 85* (6), 1359-67. https:// doi.org/10.1046/j.1471-4159.2003.01706.x. https:// www.ncbi.nlm.nih. gov/pubmed/12787055.

Delnomdedieu, M. (2018). "PDE10i and HD: Learnings from the Amaryllis studies." *CHDI's 13th Annual HD Therapeutics Conference,* 2018, Palm Springs. Accessed 08/10/2019. https:// chdifoundation.org/2018-conference/#delnomdedieu.

Delnomdedieu, M., Tan, Y., Ogden, A., Berger, Z. & Reilmann, R. (2018). "A randomized, double-blind, placebo-controlled phase ii efficacy and safety study of the PDE10A inhibitor PF-02545920 in huntington disease (amaryllis)." *J Neurol Neurosurg Psychiatry, 89,* no. Suppl 1 A99-A100.

DiFiglia, M., Sena-Esteves, M., Chase, K., Sapp, E., Pfister, E., Sass, M., Yoder, J., Reeves, P., Pandey, R. K., Rajeev, K. G., Manoharan, M., Sah, D. W., Zamore, P. D. & Aronin, N. (2007). "Therapeutic silencing of mutant huntingtin with siRNA attenuates striatal and cortical neuropathology and behavioral deficits." *Proc Natl Acad Sci USA, 104* (43), 17204-9. https://doi.org/10.1073/pnas.0708285104. https://www.ncbi.nlm.nih.gov/pubmed/17940007.

Ehrnhoefer, D. E., Caron, N. S., Deng, Y., Qiu, X., Tsang, M. & Hayden, M. R. (2016). "Laquinimod decreases Bax expression and reduces caspase-6 activation in neurons." *Exp Neurol, 283* (Pt A), 121-8. https://doi.org/10.1016/j.expneurol.2016.06.008. https://www. ncbi.nlm.nih.gov/pubmed/27296315.

Fekete, R., Davidson, A. & Jankovic, J. (2012). "Clinical assessment of the effect of tetrabenazine on functional scales in huntington disease: a pilot open label study." *Tremor Other Hyperkinet Mov (N Y), 2.* https://doi.org/10.7916/D8DN43SC. https://www.ncbi.nlm.nih.gov/ pubmed/23439575.

Frank, S. (2009). "Tetrabenazine as anti-chorea therapy in Huntington disease: an open-label continuation study. Huntington Study Group/TETRA-HD Investigators." *BMC Neurol, 9,* 62. https:// doi.org/10.1186/1471-2377-9-62. https://www.ncbi.nlm.nih.gov/pub med/20021666.

Frank, S., Ondo, W., Fahn, S., Hunter, C., Oakes, D., Plumb, S., Marshall, F., Shoulson, I., Eberly, S., Walker, F., Factor, S., Hunt, V., Shinaman, A. & Jankovic, J. (2008). "A study of chorea after tetrabenazine withdrawal in patients with Huntington disease." *Clin Neuropharmacol, 31* (3), 127-33. https://doi.org/10.1097/ WNF.0b013e3180ca77ea. https://www.ncbi.nlm.nih.gov/ pubmed/ 18520979.

Frank, S., Stamler, D., Kayson, E., Claassen, D. O., Colcher, A., Davis, C., Duker, A., Eberly, S., Elmer, L., Furr-Stimming, E., Gudesblatt, M., Hunter, C., Jankovic, J., Kostyk, S. K., Kumar, R., Loy, C., Mallonee, W., Oakes, D., Scott, B. L., Sung, V., Goldstein, J., Vaughan, C., Testa, C. M. & Investigators Huntington Study Group/Alternatives for Reducing Chorea in Huntington Disease. (2017). "Safety of Converting From Tetrabenazine to Deutetrabenazine for the Treatment of Chorea." *JAMA Neurol, 74* (8), 977-982. https://doi.org/10.1001/ jamaneurol.2017.1352. http://www.ncbi.nlm.nih.gov/pubmed/28692 723.

Garcia-Miralles, M., Geva, M., Tan, Nabm Yusof, J. Y., Cha, Y., Kusko, R., Tan, L. J., Xu, X., Grossman, I., Orbach, A., Hayden, M. R. & Pouladi, M. A. (2017). "Early pridopidine treatment improves behavioral and transcriptional deficits in YAC128 Huntington disease mice." *JCI Insight*, 2 (23). https://doi.org/10.1172/jci.insight.95665. https://www. ncbi.nlm.nih.gov/pubmed/29212949.

Garcia-Miralles, M., Hong, X., Tan, L. J., Caron, N. S., Huang, Y., To, X. V., Lin, R. Y., Franciosi, S., Papapetropoulos, S., Hayardeny, L., Hayden, M. R., Chuang, K. H. & Pouladi, M. A. (2016). "Laquinimod rescues striatal, cortical and white matter pathology and results in modest behavioural improvements in the YAC128 model of Huntington disease." *Sci Rep*, *6*, 31652. https://doi.org/ 10.1038/ srep31652. http://www.ncbi.nlm.nih.gov/pubmed/27528441.

Gelderblom, H., Wustenberg, T., McLean, T., Mutze, L., Fischer, W., Saft, C., Hoffmann, R., Sussmuth, S., Schlattmann, P., van Duijn, E., Landwehrmeyer, B. & Priller, J. (2017). "Bupropion for the treatment of apathy in Huntington's disease: A multicenter, randomised, double-blind, placebo-controlled, prospective crossover trial." *PLoS One*, *12* (3), e0173872. https://doi.org/10.1371/journal.pone.0173872. https:// www.ncbi.nlm.nih.gov/pubmed/28323838.

Granic, I., Lobel, A. & Engels, R. C. (2014). "The benefits of playing video games." *Am Psychol*, *69* (1), 66-78. https://doi.org/ 10.1037/a0034857. https://www.ncbi.nlm.nih.gov/pubmed/24295515.

Hersch, S. & Huntington Study Group. (2008). "PHEND-HD: A Safety, Tolerability, and Biomarker Study of Phenylbutyrate in Symptomatic HD." *Neurotherapeutics*, *5* (2), 363.

Hersch, S. M., Gevorkian, S., Marder, K., Moskowitz, C., Feigin, A., Cox, M., Como, P., Zimmerman, C., Lin, M., Zhang, L., Ulug, A. M., Beal, M. F., Matson, W., Bogdanov, M., Ebbel, E., Zaleta, A., Kaneko, Y., Jenkins, B., Hevelone, N., Zhang, H., Yu, H., Schoenfeld, D., Ferrante, R. & Rosas, H. D. (2006). "Creatine in Huntington disease is safe, tolerable, bioavailable in brain and reduces serum 8OH2'dG." *Neurology*, *66* (2), 250-2. https://doi.org/10.1212/ 01.wnl.0000 194318.74946.b6. https:// www.ncbi.nlm.nih.gov/ pubmed/16434666.

Hersch, S. M., Schifitto, G., Oakes, D., Bredlau, A. L., Meyers, C. M., Nahin, R., Rosas, H. D., Crest, E. & Investigators Huntington Study Group, and Coordinators. (2017). "The CREST-E study of creatine for

Huntington disease: A randomized controlled trial." *Neurology, 89* (6), 594-601. https://doi.org/10.1212/WNL.0000000000004209. https:// www.ncbi.nlm.nih.gov/pubmed/28701493.

Horizon Investigators of the Huntington Study Group, and European Huntington's Disease Network. (2013). "A randomized, double-blind, placebo-controlled study of latrepirdine in patients with mild to moderate Huntington disease." *JAMA Neurol, 70* (1), 25-33. https:// doi.org/10.1001/2013.jamaneurol.382. https:// www.ncbi.nlm.nih.gov/ pubmed/23108692.

Huntington Study Group. (2004). "Minocycline safety and tolerability in Huntington disease." *Neurology, 63* (3), 547-9. https://doi.org/10.1212/ 01.wnl.0000133403.30559.ff. https://www.ncbi.nlm.nih.gov/ pubmed/ 15304592.

Huntington Study Group. (2006). "Tetrabenazine as antichorea therapy in Huntington disease: a randomized controlled trial." *Neurology, 66* (3), 366-72. https:// doi.org/10.1212/01.wnl.0000198586.85250.13. https:// www.ncbi.nlm. nih.gov/pubmed/16476934.

Huntington Study Group. (2008). "Randomized controlled trial of ethyl-eicosapentaenoic acid in Huntington disease: the TREND-HD study." *Arch Neurol, 65* (12), 1582-9. https://doi.org/10.1001/ archneur.65.12.1582. https://www.ncbi.nlm.nih.gov/pubmed/19064 745.

Huntington Study Group, Frank, S., Testa, C. M., Stamler, D., Kayson, E., Davis, C., Edmondson, M. C., Kinel, S., Leavitt, B., Oakes, D., O'Neill, C., Vaughan, C., Goldstein, J., Herzog, M., Snively, V., Whaley, J., Wong, C., Suter, G., Jankovic, J., Jimenez-Shahed, J., Hunter, C., Claassen, D. O., Roman, O. C., Sung, V., Smith, J., Janicki, S., Clouse, R., Saint-Hilaire, M., Hohler, A., Turpin, D., James, R. C., Rodriguez, R., Rizer, K., Anderson, K. E., Heller, H., Carlson, A., Criswell, S., Racette, B. A., Revilla, F. J., Nucifora, F., Jr. Margolis, R. L., Ong, M., Mendis, T., Mendis, N., Singer, C., Quesada, M., Paulsen, J. S., Brashers-Krug, T., Miller, A., Kerr, J., Dubinsky, R. M., Gray, C., Factor, S. A., Sperin, E., Molho, E.,, Eglow, M., Evans, S., Kumar, R., Reeves, C., Samii, A., Chouinard, S., Beland, M., Scott, B. L., Hickey,

P. T., Esmail, S., Fung, W. L., Gibbons, C., Qi, L., Colcher, A., Hackmyer, C., McGarry, A., Klos, K., Gudesblatt, M., Fafard, L., Graffitti, L., Schneider, D. P., Dhall, R., Wojcieszek, J. M., LaFaver, K., Duker, A., Neefus, E., Wilson-Perez, H., Shprecher, D., Wall, P., Blindauer, K. A., Wheeler, L., Boyd, J. T., Houston, E., Farbman, E. S., Agarwal, P., Eberly, S. W., Watts, A., Tariot, P. N., Feigin, A., Evans, S., Beck, C., Orme, C., Edicola, J. & Christopher, E. (2016). "Effect of Deutetrabenazine on Chorea Among Patients With Huntington Disease: A Randomized Clinical Trial." *JAMA, 316* (1), 40-50. https:// doi.org/ 10.1001/jama.2016.8655.   http://www.ncbi.nlm.nih.gov/pubmed/2738 0342.

Huntington Study Group, Domino Investigators. (2010). "A futility study of minocycline in Huntington's disease." *Mov Disord, 25* (13), 2219-24. https://doi.org/10.1002/mds.23236.   https://www.ncbi.nlm.nih.gov/ pubmed/20721920.

Huntington Study Group, Hart Investigators. (2013). "A randomized, double-blind, placebo-controlled trial of pridopidine in Huntington's disease." *Mov Disord, 28* (10), 1407-15. https://doi.org/ 10.1002/mds.25362. https://www.ncbi.nlm.nih.gov/pubmed/23450660.

Huntington Study Group Reach. H. D. Investigators. (2015). "Safety, tolerability, and efficacy of PBT2 in Huntington's disease: a phase 2, randomised, double-blind, placebo-controlled trial." *Lancet Neurol, 14* (1), 39-47. https://doi.org/10.1016/S1474-4422(14)70262-5. https://www.ncbi.nlm.nih.gov/pubmed/25467848.

Hyson, C., Oliva, R., LaDonna, K. A., Akwaa, F., Richards, J. & Sahler, O. J. (2005). "A pilot study of music therapy in Huntington's disease." *J Neurol Neurosurg Psychiatry, 76*, no. Suppl 4, A29.

Jankovic, J. & Orman, J. (1988). "Tetrabenazine therapy of dystonia, chorea, tics, and other dyskinesias." *Neurology, 38* (3), 391-4. https:// doi.org/10.1212/wnl.38.3.391. https://www.ncbi.nlm.nih.gov/ pubmed/ 3279337.

Kegelmeyer, D. A., Kloos, A. D., Fritz, N. E., Fiumedora, M. M., White, S. E. & Kostyk, S. K. (2014). "Impact of tetrabenazine on gait and functional mobility in individuals with Huntington's disease." *J Neurol*

Sci, *347* (1-2), 219-23. https://doi.org/10.1016/j.jns.2014.09.053. https://www.ncbi.nlm.nih.gov/pubmed/25456459.

Kieburtz, K., McDermott, M. P., Voss, T. S., Corey-Bloom, J., Deuel, L. M., Dorsey, E. R., Factor, S., Geschwind, M. D., Hodgeman, K., Kayson, E., Noonberg, S., Pourfar, M., Rabinowitz, K., Ravina, B., Sanchez-Ramos, J., Seely, L., Walker, F. A. & Feigin, Group Dimebon in Subjects with Huntington Disease Investigators of the Huntington Study, and Dimond Investigators Huntington Disease Study Group. (2010). "A randomized, placebo-controlled trial of latrepirdine in Huntington disease." *Arch Neurol*, *67* (2), 154-60. https://doi.org/ 10.1001/archneurol.2009.334. https://www.ncbi.nlm.nih.gov/ pubmed/ 20142523.

Kloos, A. D., Fritz, N. E., Kostyk, S. K., Young, G. S. & Kegelmeyer, D. A. (2013). "Video game play (Dance Dance Revolution) as a potential exercise therapy in Huntington's disease: a controlled clinical trial." *Clin Rehabil*, *27* (11), 972-82. https://doi.org/10.1177/ 0269 215513487235. https://www.ncbi.nlm.nih.gov/pubmed/23787940.

Kusko, R., Dreymann, J., Ross, J., Cha, Y., Escalante-Chong, R., Garcia-Miralles, M., Tan, L. J., Burczynski, M. E., Zeskind, B., Laifenfeld, D., Pouladi, M., Geva, M., Grossman, I. & Hayden, M. R. (2018). "Large-scale transcriptomic analysis reveals that pridopidine reverses aberrant gene expression and activates neuroprotective pathways in the YAC128 HD mouse." *Mol Neurodegener*, *13* (1), 25. https://doi.org/10.1186/ s13024-018-0259-3. https://www.ncbi.nlm.nih.gov/pubmed/29783994.

La Spada, A. R., Weydt, P. & Pineda, V. V. (2011). "Huntington's Disease Pathogenesis: Mechanisms and Pathways." In *Neurobiology of Huntington's Disease: Applications to Drug Discovery*, edited by D. C. Lo and R. E. Hughes, In Frontiers in Neuroscience. Boca Raton (FL).

Landwehrmeyer, G. B., Dubois, B., de Yebenes, J. G., Kremer, B., Gaus, W., Kraus, P. H., Przuntek, H., Dib, M., Doble, A., Fischer, W., Ludolph, A. C. & Group European Huntington's Disease Initiative Study. (2007). "Riluzole in Huntington's disease: a 3-year, randomized controlled study." *Ann Neurol*, *62* (3), 262-72. https://doi.org/10.1002/ ana.21181. https://www.ncbi.nlm.nih.gov/pubmed/17702031.

Li, C., Yuan, K. & Schluesener, H. (2013). "Impact of minocycline on neurodegenerative diseases in rodents: a meta-analysis." *Rev Neurosci, 24* (5), 553-62. https://doi.org/10.1515/revneuro-2013-0040. https://www.ncbi.nlm.nih.gov/pubmed/24077620.

Lopez-Sendon Moreno, J. L., Garcia Caldentey, J., Trigo Cubillo, P., Ruiz Romero, C., Garcia Ribas, G., Alonso Arias, M. A., Garcia de Yebenes, M. J., Tolon, R. M., Galve-Roperh, I., Sagredo, O., Valdeolivas, S., Resel, E., Ortega-Gutierrez, S., Garcia-Bermejo, M. L., Fernandez Ruiz, J., Guzman, M. & Garcia de Yebenes Prous, J. (2016). "A double-blind, randomized, cross-over, placebo-controlled, pilot trial with Sativex in Huntington's disease." *J Neurol, 263* (7), 1390-400. https://doi.org/10.1007/s00415-016-8145-9. https:// www.ncbi.nlm.nih.gov/pubmed/27159993.

Lucetti, C., Gambaccini, G., Bernardini, S., Dell'Agnello, G., Petrozzi, L., Rossi, G., Bonuccelli, U. (2002). "Amantadine in Huntington's disease: open-label video-blinded study." *Neurol Sci. 23* (Suppl 2), S83-4. https://doi.org/10.1007/s100720200081. https://www.ncbi.nlm.nih.gov/pubmed/ 12548355

McBride, J. L., Boudreau, R. L., Harper, S. Q., Staber, P. D., Monteys, A. M., Martins, I., Gilmore, B. L., Burstein, H., Peluso, R. W., Polisky, B., Carter, B. J. & Davidson, B. L. (2008). "Artificial miRNAs mitigate shRNA-mediated toxicity in the brain: implications for the therapeutic development of RNAi." *Proc Natl Acad Sci U S A, 105* (15), 5868-73. https://doi.org/10.1073/pnas.0801775105. https:// www.ncbi.nlm.nih.gov/pubmed/18398004.

McGarry, A., Kieburtz, K., Abler, V., Grachev, I. D., Gandhi, S., Auinger, P., Papapetropoulos, S. & Hayden, M. (2017). "Safety and Exploratory Efficacy at 36 Months in Open-HART, an Open-Label Extension Study of Pridopidine in Huntington's Disease." *J Huntingtons Dis, 6* (3), 189-199. https://doi.org/10.3233/JHD-170241. https://www.ncbi.nlm.nih.gov/pubmed/28826192.

McGarry, A., McDermott, M., Kieburtz, K., de Blieck, E. A., Beal, F., Marder, K., Ross, C., Shoulson, I., Gilbert, P., Mallonee, W. M., Guttman, M., Wojcieszek, J., Kumar, R., LeDoux, M. S., Jenkins, M.,

Rosas, H. D., Nance, M., Biglan, K., Como, P., Dubinsky, R. M., Shannon, K. M., O'Suilleabhain, P., Chou, K., Walker, F., Martin, W., Wheelock, V. L., McCusker, E., Jankovic, J., Singer, C., Sanchez-Ramos, J., Scott, B., Suchowersky, O., Factor, S. A., Higgins, D. S., Jr. Molho, E., Revilla, F., Caviness, J. N., Friedman, J. H., Perlmutter, J. S., Feigin, A., Anderson, K., Rodriguez, R., McFarland, N. R., Margolis, R. L., Farbman, E. S., Raymond, L. A., Suski, V., Kostyk, S., Colcher, A., Seeberger, L., Epping, E., Esmail, S., Diaz, N., Fung, W. L., Diamond, A., Frank, S., Hanna, P., Hermanowicz, N., Dure, L. S., Cudkowicz, M. & Care Investigators Huntington Study Group, and Coordinators. (2017). "A randomized, double-blind, placebo-controlled trial of coenzyme Q10 in Huntington disease." *Neurology*, *88* (2), 152-159. https://doi.org/10.1212/WNL.0000000000003478. https://www.ncbi.nlm.nih.gov/pubmed/27913695.

Mestre, T. A. (2019). "Recent advances in the therapeutic development for Huntington disease." *Parkinsonism Relat Disord*, *59*, 125-130. https://doi.org/10.1016/j.parkreldis.2018.12.003. https://www.ncbi.nlm.nih.gov/pubmed/30616867.

Mestre, T., Ferreira, J., Coelho, M. M., Rosa, M. & Sampaio, C. (2009). "Therapeutic interventions for symptomatic treatment in Huntington's disease." *Cochrane Database Syst Rev*, (3), CD006456. https://doi.org/10.1002/14651858.CD006456.pub2. https://www.ncbi.nlm.nih.gov/pubmed/19588393.

Mueller, S. M., Gehrig, S. M., Petersen, J. A., Frese, S., Mihaylova, V., Ligon-Auer, M., Khmara, N., Nuoffer, J. M., Schaller, A., Lundby, C., Toigo, M. & Jung, H. H. (2017). "Effects of endurance training on skeletal muscle mitochondrial function in Huntington disease patients." *Orphanet J Rare Dis*, *12* (1), 184. https://doi.org/ 10.1186/s13023-017-0740-z. https://www.ncbi.nlm.nih.gov/pubmed/ 29258585.

Musumeci, O., Naini, A., Slonim, A. E., Skavin, N., Hadjigeorgiou, G. L., Krawiecki, N., Weissman, B. M., Tsao, C. Y., Mendell, J. R., Shanske, S., De Vivo, D. C., Hirano, M. & DiMauro, S. (2001). "Familial cerebellar ataxia with muscle coenzyme Q10 deficiency." *Neurology*, *56*

(7), 849-55. https://doi.org/10.1212/wnl.56.7.849. https:// www.ncbi. nlm.nih.gov/pubmed/11294920.

O'Suilleabhain, P. & Dewey, R. B. Jr. (2003). "A randomized trial of amantadine in Huntington disease." *Arch Neurol, 60* (7), 996-8. https://doi.org/10.1001/archneur.60.7.996. https:// www.ncbi.nlm.nih. gov/pubmed/12873857.

Pallos, J., Bodai, L., Lukacsovich, T., Purcell, J. M., Steffan, J. S., Thompson, L. M. & Marsh, J. L. (2008). "Inhibition of specific HDACs and sirtuins suppresses pathogenesis in a Drosophila model of Huntington's disease." *Hum Mol Genet, 17* (23), 3767-75. https:// doi.org/10.1093/hmg/ddn273. https://www.ncbi.nlm.nih.gov/ pubmed/ 18762557.

Pepping, J. (1999). "Coenzyme Q10." *Am J Health Syst Pharm* 56 (6): 519-21. https://doi.org/10.1093/ajhp/56.6.519. https:// www.ncbi.nlm.nih. gov/pubmed/10192685.

Pfister, E. L., DiNardo, N., Mondo, E., Borel, F., Conroy, F., Fraser, C., Gernoux, G., Han, X., Hu, D., Johnson, E., Kennington, L., Liu, P., Reid, S. J., Sapp, E., Vodicka, P., Kuchel, T., Morton, A. J., Howland, D., Moser, R., Sena-Esteves, M., Gao, G., Mueller, C., DiFiglia, M. & Aronin, N. (2018). "Artificial miRNAs Reduce Human Mutant Huntingtin Throughout the Striatum in a Transgenic Sheep Model of Huntington's Disease." *Hum Gene Ther, 29* (6), 663-673. https:// doi.org/10.1089/hum.2017.199.   https://www.ncbi.nlm.nih.gov/pub med/29207890.

Reilmann, R., Squitieri, F., Priller, J., Saft, C., Mariotti, C., Suessmuth, S. D., Nemeth, A., Tabrizi, S., Quarrell, O., Craufurd, D., Rickards, H., Rosser, A., Borje, D., Michaela, T., Angieszka, S., Fischer, D., Macdonald, D., Munoz-Sanjuan, I., Pacifici, R., Frost, C., Farmer, R., Landwehrmeyer, B. & Westerberg, G. (2014). "Safety and Tolerability of Selisistat for the Treatment of Huntington's Disease: Results from a Randomized, Double-Blind, Placebo-Controlled Phase II Trial (S47.004)." *Neurology, 82,* no. Suppl 10.

Reilmann, R., McGarry, A., Grachev, I. D., Savola, J. M., Borowsky, B., Eyal, E., Gross, N., Langbehn, D., Schubert, R., Wickenberg, A. T.,

Papapetropoulos, S., Hayden, M., Squitieri, F., Kieburtz, K., Landwehrmeyer, G. B. & Network European Huntington's Disease, and investigators Huntington Study Group. (2019). "Safety and efficacy of pridopidine in patients with Huntington's disease (PRIDE-HD): a phase 2, randomised, placebo-controlled, multicentre, dose-ranging study." *Lancet Neurol*, *18* (2), 165-176. https://doi.org/ 10.1016/S1474-4422(18)30391-0. https:// www.ncbi.nlm.nih.gov/pubmed/30563778.

Reilmann, R., Rouzade-Dominguez, M. L., Saft, C., Sussmuth, S. D., Priller, J., Rosser, A., Rickards, H., Schols, L., Pezous, N., Gasparini, F., Johns, D., Landwehrmeyer, G. B. & Gomez-Mancilla, B. (2015). "A randomized, placebo-controlled trial of AFQ056 for the treatment of chorea in Huntington's disease." *Mov Disord*, *30* (3), 427-31. https://doi.org/10.1002/mds.26174. https://www.ncbi.nlm.nih.gov/ pubmed/25689146.

Rodrigues, F. B., Quinn, L. & Wild, E. J. (2019). "Huntington's Disease Clinical Trials Corner: January 2019." *J Huntingtons Dis*, *8* (1), 115-125. https://doi.org/10.3233/JHD-190001. https://www.ncbi.nlm.nih. gov/pubmed/30776019.

Rosas, H. D., Doros, G., Gevorkian, S., Malarick, K., Reuter, M., Coutu, J. P., Triggs, T. D., Wilkens, P. J., Matson, W., Salat, D. H. & Hersch, S. M. (2014). "PRECREST: a phase II prevention and biomarker trial of creatine in at-risk Huntington disease." *Neurology*, *82* (10), 850-7. https://doi.org/10.1212/WNL.0000000000000187. https://www.ncbi.nlm.nih.gov/pubmed/24510496.

Ross, C. A., Aylward, E. H., Wild, E. J., Langbehn, D. R., Long, J. D., Warner, J. H., Scahill, R. I., Leavitt, B. R., Stout, J. C., Paulsen, J. S., Reilmann, R., Unschuld, P. G., Wexler, A., Margolis, R. L. & Tabrizi, S. J. (2014). "Huntington disease: natural history, biomarkers and prospects for therapeutics." *Nat Rev Neurol*, *10* (4), 204-16. https:// doi.org/10.1038/nrneurol.2014.24. http://www.ncbi.nlm.nih.gov/ pub med/24614516.

Ross, C., Biglan, K., Killoran, A., Beal, M. F., Matson, W., Julian-Baros, E., Yoritomo, N., Gao, S., McDermott, M. & Huntington Study Group PREQUEL Investigators. (2014). "PREQUEL—A Multicenter Phase II

Study of Coenzyme Q10 in PreManifest Huntington Disease." *Neurotherapeutics*, *11*, 214.

Sadeghi, M., Barlow-Krelina, E., Gibbons, C., Shaikh, K. T., Fung, W. L. A., Meschino, W. S. & Till, C. (2017). "Feasibility of computerized working memory training in individuals with Huntington disease." *PLoS One*, *12* (4), e0176429. https://doi.org/10.1371/ journal.pone.0176429. https://www.ncbi.nlm.nih.gov/pubmed/ 28453532.

Schiefer, J., Landwehrmeyer, G. B., Luesse, H. G., Sprunken, A., Puls, C., Milkereit, A., Milkereit, E. & Kosinski, C. M. (2002). "Riluzole prolongs survival time and alters nuclear inclusion formation in a transgenic mouse model of Huntington's disease." *Mov Disord*, *17* (4), 748-57. https://doi.org/10.1002/mds.10229. https:// www.ncbi.nlm.nih. gov/pubmed/12210870.

Schulte, J. & Littleton, J. T. (2011). "The biological function of the Huntingtin protein and its relevance to Huntington's Disease pathology." *Curr Trends Neurol*, *5*, 65-78. https:// www.ncbi.nlm.nih. gov/pubmed/22180703.

Shin, J. W., Kim, K. H., Chao, M. J., Atwal, R. S., Gillis, T., MacDonald, M. E., Gusella, J. F. & Lee, J. M. (2016). "Permanent inactivation of Huntington's disease mutation by personalized allele-specific CRISPR/Cas9." *Hum Mol Genet*, *25* (20), 4566-4576. https://doi.org/ 10.1093/hmg/ddw286. https://www.ncbi.nlm.nih.gov/pubmed/ 28172 889.

Smith, E. S., Jonason, A., Reilly, C., Veeraraghavan, J., Fisher, T., Doherty, M., Klimatcheva, E., Mallow, C., Cornelius, C., Leonard, J. E., Marchi, N., Janigro, D., Argaw, A. T., Pham, T., Seils, J., Bussler, H., Torno, S., Kirk, R., Howell, A., Evans, E. E., Paris, M., Bowers, W. J., John, G. & Zauderer, M. (2015). "SEMA4D compromises blood-brain barrier, activates microglia, and inhibits remyelination in neurodegenerative disease." *Neurobiol Dis*, *73*, 254-68. https:// doi.org/10.1016/ j.nbd.2014.10.008. https:// www.ncbi.nlm.nih.gov/ pubmed/25461192.

Smith, M. R., Syed, A., Lukacsovich, T., Purcell, J., Barbaro, B. A., Worthge, S. A., Wei, S. R., Pollio, G., Magnoni, L., Scali, C., Massai, L., Franceschini, D., Camarri, M., Gianfriddo, M., Diodato, E., Thomas, R., Gokce, O., Tabrizi, S. J., Caricasole, A., Landwehrmeyer, B., Menalled, L., Murphy, C., Ramboz, S., Luthi-Carter, R., Westerberg, G. & Marsh, J. L. (2014). "A potent and selective Sirtuin 1 inhibitor alleviates pathology in multiple animal and cell models of Huntington's disease." *Hum Mol Genet*, *23* (11), 2995-3007. https:// doi.org/10.1093/ hmg/ddu010. https://www.ncbi.nlm.nih.gov/ pubmed/ 24436303.

Southwell, A. L., Franciosi, S., Villanueva, E. B., Xie, Y., Winter, L. A., Veeraraghavan, J., Jonason, A., Felczak, B., Zhang, W., Kovalik, V., Waltl, S., Hall, G., Pouladi, M. A., Smith, E. S., Bowers, W. J., Zauderer, M. & Hayden, M. R. (2015). "Anti-semaphorin 4D immunotherapy ameliorates neuropathology and some cognitive impairment in the YAC128 mouse model of Huntington disease." *Neurobiol Dis*, *76*, 46-56. https://doi.org/10.1016/j.nbd.2015.01.002. http://www.ncbi.nlm.nih.gov/pubmed/25662335.

Squitieri, F., Di Pardo, A., Favellato, M., Amico, E., Maglione, V. & Frati, L. (2015). "Pridopidine, a dopamine stabilizer, improves motor performance and shows neuroprotective effects in Huntington disease R6/2 mouse model." *J Cell Mol Med*, *19* (11), 2540-8. https:// doi.org/10.1111/jcmm.12604. https://www.ncbi.nlm.nih.gov/ pubmed/ 26094900.

Stanek, L. M., Sardi, S. P., Mastis, B., Richards, A. R., Treleaven, C. M., Taksir, T., Misra, K., Cheng, S. H. & Shihabuddin, L. S. (2014). "Silencing mutant huntingtin by adeno-associated virus-mediated RNA interference ameliorates disease manifestations in the YAC128 mouse model of Huntington's disease." *Hum Gene Ther*, *25* (5), 461-74. https://doi.org/10.1089/hum.2013.200. https://www.ncbi.nlm.nih.gov/ pubmed/24484067.

Stanek, L. M., Yang, W., Angus, S., Sardi, P. S., Hayden, M. R., Hung, G. H., Bennett, C. F., Cheng, S. H. & Shihabuddin, L. S. (2013). "Antisense oligonucleotide-mediated correction of transcriptional dysregulation is correlated with behavioral benefits in the YAC128 mouse model of Huntington's disease." *J Huntingtons Dis*, 2 (2), 217-28. https:// doi.org/ 10.3233/ JHD-130057. https://www.ncbi.nlm.nih.gov/pubmed/ 25063 516.

Stefanko, D. P., Shah, V. D., Yamasaki, W. K., Petzinger, G. M. & Jakowec, M. W. (2017). "Treadmill exercise delays the onset of non-motor behaviors and striatal pathology in the CAG140 knock-in mouse model of Huntington's disease." *Neurobiol Dis*, *105*, 15-32. https:// doi.org/10.1016/j.nbd.2017.05.004. https://www.ncbi.nlm.nih.gov/ pubmed/28502806.

Stocchi, F., Rascol, O., Destee, A., Hattori, N., Hauser, R. A., Lang, A. E., Poewe, W., Stacy, M., Tolosa, E., Gao, H., Nagel, J., Merschhemke, M., Graf, A., Kenney, C. & Trenkwalder, C. (2013). "AFQ056 in Parkinson patients with levodopa-induced dyskinesia: 13-week, randomized, dose-finding study." *Mov Disord*, *28* (13), 1838-46. https://doi.org/10. 1002/mds.25561. https:// www.ncbi.nlm.nih.gov/ pubmed/23853029.

Sussmuth, S. D., Haider, S., Landwehrmeyer, G. B., Farmer, R., Frost, C., Tripepi, G., Andersen, C. A., Di Bacco, M., Lamanna, C., Diodato, E., Massai, L., Diamanti, D., Mori, E., Magnoni, L., Dreyhaupt, J., Schiefele, K., Craufurd, D., Saft, C., Rudzinska, M., Ryglewicz, D., Orth, M., Brzozy, S., Baran, A., Pollio, G., Andre, R., Tabrizi, S. J., Darpo, B., Westerberg, G. & Paddington Consortium. (2015). "An exploratory double-blind, randomized clinical trial with selisistat, a SirT1 inhibitor, in patients with Huntington's disease." *Br J Clin Pharmacol*, *79* (3), 465-76. https://doi.org/10.1111/bcp.12512. https:// www.ncbi.nlm.nih.gov/pubmed/25223731.

Tabrizi, S. J., Ghosh, R. & Leavitt, B. R. (2019). "Huntingtin Lowering Strategies for Disease Modification in Huntington's Disease." *Neuron*, *102* (4), 899. https://doi.org/10.1016/j.neuron.2019.05.001. https:// www.ncbi.nlm.nih.gov/pubmed/31121127.

Tabrizi, S. J., Leavitt, B. R., Landwehrmeyer, G. B., Wild, E. J., Saft, C., Barker, R. A., Blair, N. F., Craufurd, D., Priller, J., Rickards, H., Rosser, A., Kordasiewicz, H. B., Czech, C., Swayze, E. E., Norris, D. A., Baumann, T., Gerlach, I., Schobel, S. A., Paz, E., Smith, A. V., Bennett, C. F. & Lane, R. M. (2019). "Targeting Huntingtin Expression in Patients with Huntington's Disease." *N Engl J Med, 380* (24), 2307-2316. https://doi.org/10.1056/NEJMoa1900907. https:// www.ncbi.nlm. nih.gov/pubmed/31059641.

Testa, C. M. & Jankovic, J. (2019). "Huntington disease: A quarter century of progress since the gene discovery." *J Neurol Sci, 396*, 52-68. https://doi.org/10.1016/j.jns.2018.09.022. https:// www.ncbi.nlm.nih. gov/pubmed/30419368.

The Huntington's Disease Collaborative Research Group. (1993). "A novel gene containing a trinucleotide repeat that is expanded and unstable on Huntington's disease chromosomes." *Cell, 72* (6), 971-83. http:// www.ncbi.nlm.nih.gov/pubmed/8458085.

Thone, J., Ellrichmann, G., Seubert, S., Peruga, I., Lee, D. H., Conrad, R., Hayardeny, L., Comi, G., Wiese, S., Linker, R. A. & Gold, R. (2012). "Modulation of autoimmune demyelination by laquinimod via induction of brain-derived neurotrophic factor." *Am J Pathol, 180* (1), 267-74. https://doi.org/10.1016/j.ajpath.2011.09.037. http:// www.ncbi.nlm. nih.gov/pubmed/22152994.

Trinkler, I., Chehere, P., Salgues, J., Monin, M. L., Tezenas du Montcel, S., Khani, S., Gargiulo, M. & Durr, A. (2019). "Contemporary Dance Practice Improves Motor Function and Body Representation in Huntington's Disease: A Pilot Study." *J Huntingtons Dis, 8* (1), 97-110. https://doi.org/10.3233/JHD-180315. https://www.ncbi.nlm.nih. gov/pubmed/30776016.

Verbessem, P., Lemiere, J., Eijnde, B. O., Swinnen, S., Vanhees, L., Van Leemputte, M., Hespel, P. & Dom, R. (2003). "Creatine supplementation in Huntington's disease: a placebo-controlled pilot trial." *Neurology, 61* (7), 925-30. https://doi.org/10.1212/ 01.wnl. 0000090629.40891.4b. https://www.ncbi.nlm.nih.gov/pubmed/ 14557 561.

Verhagen Metman L., Morris, M.J., Farmer, C., Gillespie, M., Mosby, K., Wuu, J., Chase, T.N. (2002). "Huntington's disease: a randomized, controlled trial using the NMDA-antagonist amantadine." *Neurology, 59* (5), 694-9. https://doi.org/10.1212/wnl.59.5.694. https://www.ncbi. nlm.nih.gov/ pubmed/12221159

Waters, S., Tedroff, J., Ponten, H., Klamer, D., Sonesson, C. & Waters, N. (2018). "Pridopidine: Overview of Pharmacology and Rationale for its Use in Huntington's Disease." *J Huntingtons Dis, 7* (1), 1-16. https:// doi.org/10.3233/JHD-170267. https://www.ncbi.nlm.nih.gov/pubmed/ 29480206.

Wild, E. J. & Tabrizi, S. J. (2014). "Targets for future clinical trials in Huntington's disease: what's in the pipeline?" *Mov Disord, 29* (11), 1434-45. https://doi.org/10.1002/mds.26007. http:// www.ncbi.nlm. nih.gov/pubmed/25155142.

Wills, A. M., Garry, J., Hubbard, J., Mezoian, T., Breen, C. T., Ortiz-Miller, C., Nalipinski, P., Sullivan, S., Berry, J. D., Cudkowicz, M., Paganoni, S., Chan, J. & Macklin, E. A. (2019). "Nutritional counseling with or without mobile health technology: a randomized open-label standard-of-care-controlled trial in ALS." *BMC Neurol, 19* (1), 104. https://doi.org/10.1186/s12883-019-1330-6. https:// www.ncbi.nlm. nih.gov/pubmed/31142272.

Wojtecki, L., Groiss, S. J., Ferrea, S., Elben, S., Hartmann, C. J., Dunnett, S. B., Rosser, A., Saft, C., Sudmeyer, M., Ohmann, C., Schnitzler, A., Vesper, J. & Network Surgical Approaches Working Group of the European Huntington's Disease. (2015). "A Prospective Pilot Trial for Pallidal Deep Brain Stimulation in Huntington's Disease." *Front Neurol, 6,* 177. https://doi.org/10.3389/fneur.2015.00177. https:// www.ncbi.nlm.nih.gov/pubmed/26347707.

Yang, S., Chang, R., Yang, H., Zhao, T., Hong, Y., Kong, H. E., Sun, X., Qin, Z., Jin, P., Li, S. & Li, X. J. (2017). "CRISPR/Cas9-mediated gene editing ameliorates neurotoxicity in mouse model of Huntington's disease." *J Clin Invest, 127* (7), 2719-2724. https:// doi.org/10. 1172/JCI92087. https://www.ncbi.nlm.nih.gov/ pubmed/ 28628038.

Yero, T. & Rey, J. A. (2008). "Tetrabenazine (Xenazine), An FDA-Approved Treatment Option For Huntington's Disease-Related Chorea." *P T*, *33* (12), 690-4. https://www.ncbi.nlm.nih.gov/pubmed/19750050.

Yhnell, E., Furby, H., Breen, R. S., Brookes-Howell, L. C., Drew, C. J. G., Playle, R., Watson, G., Metzler-Baddeley, C., Rosser, A. E. & Busse, M. E. (2018). "Exploring computerised cognitive training as a therapeutic intervention for people with Huntington's disease (CogTrainHD): protocol for a randomised feasibility study." *Pilot Feasibility Stud*, *4*, 45. https://doi.org/10.1186/s40814-018-0237-0. https://www.ncbi.nlm.nih.gov/pubmed/29445514.

In: Living with Huntington's Disease ISBN: 978-1-53616-729-0
Editor: Sherman Howell © 2020 Nova Science Publishers, Inc.

Chapter 3

EMOTIONAL AND COMMUNICATIONAL ISSUES IN HUNTINGTON'S DISEASE

*Roman Adamczyk**

Institute of Nursing, Faculty of Public Policies in Opava,
Opava, Czech Republic

ABSTRACT

Huntington's disease is a devastating neurological disorder impacting all aspects of individual functioning, including cognition, mood, self-care, social interaction and the capacity for work. Similarly to other patients with neurodegenerative diseases, Huntington sufferers face innumerable problems in everyday life, both within their bodies and psyches, and in the natural and social environments. The following chapter centers on emotional and communicational issues in Huntington's disease and their interrelations, covering a range of topics from depressive symptomatology, anxiety, helplessness or anger, to verbal and non-verbal communication and assistive technology. As the communication processes get increasingly disrupted during disease progression, knowing what the patient feels and needs represents a major challenge for both professional and lay caregivers. Simultaneously, the emotional stratum of a Huntington

* Corresponding Author's E-mail: roman.adamczyk@fvp.slu.cz.

patient's personality is subject to various independent detrimental effects unrelated to communication. An overview of current research combined with personal stories is provided in the present chapter along with discussion of emotional suffering of all persons involved.

Keywords: Huntington's disease, emotion, psychiatric disorder, communication

INTRODUCTION

The name of Huntington's disease, an entity closely linked to mutations causing aberrant huntingtin protein production, is based on eponymic reference to George Huntington, an American physician, who concisely described (in 1872, at the age of 21) the clinical presentation of this nosological unit. Huntington had been a keen observer as early as his childhood years, accompanying his father on medical rounds (Durbach and Hayden 1993). Thanks to his long-term efforts and thanks to contributions of successive generations with many other excellent minds in medical sciences, the body of knowledge about the disease has increased significantly.

Almost 150 years of Huntington's disease research, however, have not yielded a definitive treatment of the disease (as is the case of many other neurodegenerative diseases). Few tangible advances have reached the patient population in terms of mitigating and/or slowing down the disease, let alone curing it. Therefore, the patients and their relatives are largely left on their own devices in fighting this abominable condition and its detrimental physical, cognitive, emotional, communicational, social and economic consequences.

The latter consequences run across the whole spectrum of the sufferer's activity and hit the very core of human identity both neurologically and psychologically, including the capacity for work, leisure, and communication. Simultaneously, Huntington's grossly disrupts the individual's emotional equilibrium. With a loss of up to 30 per cent of brain weight and an average of 22 per cent of cerebral cortex volume,

Huntington's disease ranks among the most devastating neurodegenerative diseases (Rüb et al. 2015; Bates, Tabrizi and Jones 2014). What is of prominent importance to the patient, however, are not the objective signs that accompany the natural history of the disease, but, rather, the impact on functioning and subjective quality of life.

EMOTIONS AND EMOTIONAL DISTURBANCES IN HUNTINGTON'S DISEASE

Traditionally, classifications of emotions as adopted over the 20th and 21st centuries, distinguish a group of emotions termed 'primary' (or, essential) on the one hand, and secondary (or, derived) on the other hand. Primary emotions are defined as those that are 'hardwired' in the brain and are direct reactions to particular stimuli (such as spotting an object that can pose danger). Contrarily, secondary emotions supersede primary emotions and are based on more elaborate pondering of either primary emotions or the complexity of situations occurring. Examples of primary, or basic, emotions in various classification systems include: 1. anger, disgust, fear, happiness, sadness, and surprise (Ekman), 2. trust (acceptance), anger, anticipation (interest), disgust, joy, fear, sadness, and surprise (Plutchick), 3. love, joy, surprise, anger, sadness, and fear (Parrots), 4. anger, fear, disgust, contempt, sadness, surprise, and joy (Humintell), 5. happiness, sadness, fear/surprise, and anger/disgust (Jack) – Meiselman 2016. Similarly, examples of secondary emotions, complex or derived, are anxiety (although it is also considered by certain scholars as a primary emotion), guilt, gratitude, hope, scorn, envy or shame (Ellis and Tucker 2015). Certain emotions can emerge as either primary, or secondary, depending on the particular situation.

Emotions in neurodegenerative disease have been studied by a number methods, including advanced imaging techniques such as functional magnetic resonance (fMRI) – Pfaff 2019. A number of abnormalities and specifics have been found in neurodegenerative disease sufferers, ranging from increased incidence of *Diagnostic and Statistical Manual (DSM)-* or

International Classification of Diseases (ICD)- classified mental disorders, through various emotional disturbances not meeting the criteria of given diagnostic units, to subjective perceptions of suffering. A systematic review of emotion recognition by leading researchers in the field indicates that recognition of facial and vocal expressions of negative emotions (including anger) tends to be impaired in Huntington patients (Henley et al. 2012). The impairment of emotion experience in Huntington's disease may involve reduction in classification accuracy (for anger, disgust, sadness and surprise as reflected in other people's facial expressions), as well as different intensity ratings compared to those of controls – elevated for certain affective scenes in experimental settings (fear, happiness) and reduced for other scenes (anger, disgust). The latter impairments seem to be closely associated with dysfunction in social interactions, which seems logical in the light of the significance of emotions in inter-human communication. – Ille et al. 2011. Further, the fact that emotional processing is affected by the disease process (possibly based on disruptions in frontostriatal pathways) seems to contribute to apathy, a frequent finding in Huntington sufferers (Osborne-Crowley et al. 2019). Although the apathetic subgroup of Huntington patients seems to have difficulty recognizing happy facial expressions, other patients may appear responsive to the latter until late stages of disease, a phenomenon confirmed by relatives who find their loved ones reacting positively to smiles and laughter.

To place the findings of emotional processing and subjective experience in a broader context, it is necessary to consider other factors, such as motor behavior and information-seeking behavior. Interestingly, Kordsachia, Labuschagne and Stout (2017) found a possible connection between visual scanning behavior and emotional alterations in Huntington's disease, with patients fixating shorter times (in a more unfocussed manner) with longer tracks on emotionally evocative natural scenes (fear, disgust, happiness, neutral, etc.) compared to controls. An eye-tracking technology was employed to assess the ocular input in this experiment. Although the interpretation of such finding is difficult, the heightened search for information observed might be a form of compensatory strategy in trying to determine the emotional valence of the pictorial stimuli presented. Reduced eye-viewing, on the other hand, might contribute to the emotion recognition deficit consistently found in clinically manifest Huntington's disease (Kordsachia, Labuschagne and Stout 2018). As cognition typically deteriorates in the disease process, evaluation of emotions based on other than self-report procedures becomes an important instrument for better insight into the emotional life of Huntington sufferers. Apart from eye-tracking, electromyography of facial muscles has been employed to detect affective abnormalities 'objectively'. A team of researchers known from the previous two studies identified diminished responses in the patient group in terms of reactions to happy and fearful faces and (consensually) disgusting scenes. Hence, it is possible to infer that both perceptive and expressive impairments may contribute to the overall picture of emotional-communicational deficit in Huntington's disease in a complex cascade of neurobiological abnormalities and social consequences. Current research suggests that subtle alterations in social cognition, including emotion recognition, may even precede the motor signs observable in manifest disease (Bora, Velakoulis and Walterfang 2016), rendering the individual more prone to social isolation early in the course of the condition. Functional magnetic resonance imaging studies seem to confirm that changes in emotional processing may be present even in pre-manifest periods, with both areas of increased activity (frontally) and decreased activity (several functional networks) in response to disgust, anger and happiness stimuli in the Ekman series (Novak et al. 2012).

As indicated, people with Huntington's disease may find it particularly difficult to identify, control or express emotions and to cope with them. Positive emotions are hard to evoke and relish for Huntington sufferers, yet any amount of positive emotions such as joy, content, or feeling of unity with others is very useful in fighting stress and despair. A variety of sources inciting desirable emotions can be employed to foster well-being, inclusive of appropriately arranged social gatherings, appetizing dishes, watching the patient's favorite comedies, or affording the patient a soft massage, if tolerated. As the disease progresses, however, experiencing positive emotions may become increasingly difficult and the emotional life of the individual may turn blunted as apathy is one of common manifestations of neurodegenerative processes and the dire situation of the sufferer, who is facing a loss of capacity for most activities and perceiving helplessness vis-à-vis the biological enemy (the disease process) inside, potentiates the overall burden. Feelings of vanity and deprivation may resurface as the sufferer loses cognitive skills, motor skills, mobility, bathroom privileges and other basic attributes of daily living. Healthy persons may be viewed as objects of envy and deterioration of one's status may result in anger or withdrawal. Preliminary research suggests that recognition of a range of positive emotions, including pleasure, from vocal, non-verbal cues is impaired in Huntington patients (Robotham et al. 2011).

Situational (short-term) emotional reactions of Huntington's sufferers may appear distinct compared to healthy controls (Quarrell 2008). Anger and irritability and their behavioral correlates, such as aggression or verbal outbursts, may become accentuated in a large proportion of patients (with prevalence reports of 38 to 73 per cent) – Paoli et al. 2017. Gradual degeneration of the caudate nucleus, an area of the cerebral striatum contributing to the inhibitory control of impulses (as well as to language communication, learning, prioritization of information and many other complex processes), appears to be a co-factor of the increased risk of bouts of anger (temper tantrums). While various studies yield somewhat divergent results, irritability and verbal outbursts seem to peak approximately 8-9 years after disease onset, although they may appear at any stage of the disease and may sometimes be marked at the beginning of the clinical course (Brandt 2018; Craufurd, Thompson and Snowden 2001). Yelling, threatening, punching and other manifestations may be the result of underlying neurodegenerative processes, yet, may also represent inner emotional states that cannot be expressed otherwise, e.g., fear, loss, frustration, discomfort, pain or feelings of hunger. While apathy, observed mainly at later stages of disease, appears to correlate with cognitive and motor decline, no such association was identified between depression and irritability features on the one hand, and severity of cognitive and motor symptoms on the other hand in a study employing the *Problem Behaviors Assessment for Huntington's Disease* (PBA-HD) – Craufurd, Thompson and Snowden 2001; Thompson et al. 2012. A number of treatment strategies have been tried for irritability in Huntington's disease, including selective serotonin reuptake inhibitors, atypical antipsychotics (especially olanzapine) or mood stabilizers (van Duijn 2010). Importantly, the social environment should be aware of the causal attribution it assumes – it is usually not the sufferer who is 'to blame' for manifestations of anger – it is the underlying disease process that cannot be averted by the patient.

In his middle-stage Huntington's disease, my loved sibling would irregularly become upset and have outbursts of anger with a hardly predictable pattern. I remember the same with my Mom, who was otherwise a very meek and friendly person. Things were thrown across the flat and shouting was 'normal' in our household. I felt that this was due to a disease process in the brain, though, in the previous generations, we did not know the 'malefactor' was Huntington's disease (diagnostics was in its infancy at that time). What is most important to me, I never blamed my Mom or my sibling for behaving that way. It was not them who initiated this. It was the odious, hated, despicable brain-damaging sickness that was behind it.

(O., a relative)

Vignette 1.

Prolonged emotional states, commonly referred to as 'mood', are subject to disruption and imbalance in many otherwise healthy individuals and in persons with a wide range of medical conditions. They may comply with the criteria of mood disorders (e.g., major depression, dysthymia, bipolar disorder) or personality disorders (such as the emotionally unstable personality disorder). If anxiety is the major feature of the individual's mindset, one of anxiety disorders may be diagnosed (e.g., generalized anxiety disorder or specific phobias). In persons with Huntington's disease, the latter disorders may occur as co-morbidities or as direct consequences of the underlying neurodegenerative disease process that affects cerebral centers of key importance for emotional processing, such as the amygdala. Abnormalities in connectivity between the amygdala (one of the number of brain regions known to lose volume during the disease process even prior to diagnosis) and the fusiform face area (responsible for identification of facial expressions of emotions in other people) have been documented by functional brain imaging and 'reading the mind in the eyes' testing, indicating emotional and related social impairment in both pre-clinical and clinical Huntington's disease (Mason et al. 2015). Moreover, the amygdala is one of the structures related to anxiety states (Ahveninen et al. 2018).

Anxiety appears to be one of the most frequent emotional/behavioral complaints of manifest Huntington sufferers, with a point prevalence ranging from 13 to 71 per cent, depending on the methods and samples used (data based on a recent systematic review by Dale and van Duijn 2015). While dysphoria, agitation, irritability and apathy appear to be similarly or even more highly prevalent (with dysphoria present in up to 70 per cent of patient populations studied – Paulsen et al. 2001), anxiety constitutes a major challenge to the inner balance of the patient and a significant stressor impacting the overall quality of life. Fear and anxiety rank among the core experiences of human existence, with fear of death, disease and disability (a cluster that we may tentatively call 'the three D's') being among the most influential (compare Freud's concept of 'thanatos'). As a disabling and disturbing emotion, prolonged anxiety hinders everyday functioning and detracts from subjective well-being. The period shortly before, during and after predictive testing for Huntington's disease in potential mutation carriers may be particularly prone to evoke anxiety, relative to the individual's expectations and test results. Further, regardless of the actual mutation status, persons at risk of Huntington's disease have increased tendency both to anxiety and hopelessness, feelings that are predictive of suicidal ideation (Anderson et al. 2016) and that should, therefore, be strictly monitored and effectively controlled by general practitioners and specialists caring for the subjects in question. The negative emotions that emerge in the course of the disease can be extremely stressful and appear to be one of the key explanations of the 4-fold to 8-fold incidence of suicidal attempts among Huntington sufferers compared to healthy controls (Bindler et al. 2010).

As research into the molecular and cellular mechanisms of Huntington's disease advances, it seems likely that anxiety and depression are somehow linked to the disruptions of normal huntingtin protein functioning (Pla et al.

2014). For the patient, however, the phenomenological, subjective aspects (including feelings) are much more important than theoretical knowledge. Anxiety as a negative emotion contributes to the complex body of suffering in Huntington's disease and it tends to be associated with depression, irritability and pain, while it does not appear to be directly linked to disease progression (Dale and van Duijn 2015). Psychosocial approaches and medication possessing anxiolytic effects, e.g., olanzapine, can be recommended by attending physicians to alleviate the symptoms of anxiety.

Depressive symptomatology, closely related to the primary emotion of sadness, is frequently found in both prodromal and manifest Huntington's disease and 33–69% of patients present with depressed mood (Epping and Paulsen 2011). Prolonged sadness, anhedonia (loss of pleasure), low self-worth, hopelessness, disrupted sleep patterns, low energy, psychomotor retardation, poor concentration, memory decline, passivity or agitation are common elements of the clinical picture of major depression (Ossig and Storch 2015). The underlying mechanisms of depression in Huntington patients are logically interpreted as a combination of the pathology related to neurodegeneration, including hypothalamic dysfunction and altered function of the Cdk5 kinase enzyme, and of emotional-social factors, such as isolation or frustration from the loss of general functioning capacity, employment or emotional bonds. Even in pre-manifest stages of the disease, i.e., before the onset of motor signs, a loss of structural connectivity in basal ganglia and an increase in functional connectivity in particular cerebral regions has been documented (McColgan et al. 2017).

Depression and associated hopelessness deserve sustained attention by medical professionals involved in Huntington patients' care for at least two reasons – the significant amount of suffering and emotional burden caused by severely dysphoric mood, and the elevated risk of suicidal ideation. Possible treatment options include counselling, psychotherapy, including cognitive-behavioral approaches, if applicable at the given stage of disease, and psychiatric medication, such as antidepressants (some of which also possess neuroprotective properties and the ability to increase brain-derived neurotrophic factor levels) or possibly lithium. Based on general assumptions respecting major depressive disorder, aerobic exercise (if viable), daylight exposure and repetitive transcranial magnetic stimulation (rTMS) may have some therapeutic potential (Davis et al. 2016). Environmental changes and mental stimulation can also prove useful in ameliorating depression in Huntington patients. Detailed monitoring of depression symptoms is also recommended in patients on tetrabenazine regimen intended to mitigate choreatic movements, although study results concerning the depressogenic effects of tetrabenazine are conflicting (Schultz et al. 2018). As Huntington's is a disease of the whole family, rather than the individual as such, it is imperative to incorporate into the treatment plan the relatives and significant others of the patient to the largest extent possible while offering enough medical, material and emotional support to prevent excessive burden on any of the parties – patients or caregivers.

Patient and expert organizations consistently emphasize the importance of emotional support in Huntington families. As the burden of disease, including the stigma of being 'salient' in various settings (e.g., when dining out, shopping, having a walk) due to chorea or other observable signs, appears severe for most patients and relatives, psychological counseling, domiciliary services and support by extended family constitute an integral part of coping. Experienced psychologists can be very helpful in analyzing the situation of the family, the inner emotional processes of the patient and opportunities for multi-faceted strategies that can mitigate the impact of disability and emotional trauma. As there exist over 600 different schools and approaches in psychotherapy (Prochaska and Norcross 2018), it can take some time to find a practitioner who will fit the needs of the sufferer and their family. For the purpose of enhancing one's balance in life under challenging circumstances set by the disease, approaches like logotherapy or existential analysis may be helpful.

Logotherapy, also called the third Viennese school of psychotherapy, was founded by psychiatrist Viktor E. Frankl following his experience in a concentration camp to help people cope with the most extreme situations of individual distress. Frankl observed that maintaining meaning in life is a crucial factor of survival. As he remarks in *Man's Search for Meaning* (Frankl 2006), reorientation toward the meaning of life can be a useful mechanism of coping with disturbing illness. Frankl has also abundantly discussed the issue of suffering, a topic profoundly represented in the lives of Huntington patients across generations. Although his discussion of this subject was not specifically directed toward patients with neurodegenerative diseases, its all-embracing character and the author's erudition in neurology allow for transposition to the area of Huntington's. Frankl repeatedly speaks of Homo patients, a suffering person, who sometimes faces an incurable disease and whose opportunity to endow meaning to his/her life is to take a brave, dignity-preserving attitude to the fateful situation (Frankl 2004).

Similarly, existential analysis, whose chief proponents were Alfried Längle and Irvin Yalom, offers a range of techniques to work with core human experience and quintessential emotions. While remaining more 'on the surface', i.e., on the behavioral level, other approaches such as cognitive behavioral therapy (CBT) may prove helpful in tackling disturbing emotions of Huntington sufferers and their caregivers. It should be noted, however, that psychological approaches are not a panacea for emotional disturbances and that other supportive measures, including medication and/or intense emotional support by family members or significant others may be necessary.

COMMUNICATIONAL ISSUES IN HUNTINGTON'S DISEASE

As indicated previously, emotions are mutually intertwined with social factors and interpersonal communication, including verbal and non-verbal, e.g., facial, messages conveyed in everyday contact between the patient and their relatives, friends and professional caregivers. Communication is generally defined as conveyance of messages between a source and a destination, e.g., a human receiver (Krauss 2001). Traditionally, communication is divided into verbal (based on spoken or written words) and non-verbal (gestures, facial expressions, body posture, distance/ proximity, smells, touch – the means of so-called tactile communication, acts or abstaining from acts – for example helping or not helping someone in a difficult situation). As such, communication serves a number of interpersonal/social purposes. In Huntington's disease, the main goal of all interventions related to communication is to enable the patient to 'stay connected' as long as possible through the development of the condition and, thus, reduce feelings of isolation and despair, as well as to keep the caregivers informed about the thoughts, needs, wishes, feelings and preferences of the subject.

> *One of the most difficult points in coping with my relative's diagnosis of Huntington's disease was the complete cessation of verbal communication after a period of broken, dysarthric speech. There were some transient attempts to bridge this communication gap by assistive technology (using a tablet), yet, due to severe chorea, the utility of this method was very limited. We were suddenly left on a speculation platform concerning the likes and dislikes, wishes and needs of our relative. That was really frustrating for both parties.*
> *(E., a family caregiver)*

Vignette 2.

Communication is based on a combination of expressive (productive) and receptive components, both of which usually become severely impaired as Huntington's disease gradually damages corresponding brain areas and specific skills. The most marked changes occur in motor coordination, resulting in manifest dysarthria. Current knowledge suggests that, unlike some other conditions, Huntington's disease does not lead to aphasic impairments but, rather, has detrimental effects on speech and writing capacity through a complex interplay of motor deterioration, including the presence of involuntary movements, and primary deficits of language and cognition. As the disease advances, handwriting becomes ragged and macrographia may occur (Phillips 1994). Speech characteristics change in line with the course of the disease and incorporate altered timing, phonation and prosody, as well as disrupted oral diadochokinesis, resulting in slurred utterances (Hartelius et al. 2003). With neostriatal pathology probably involved, the neurolinguistic abnormalities observed include word-finding difficulties, paraphasic errors, diminished levels of syntactic complexity and overall lexical production, along with reductions in phrase/sentence length and articulatory agility. The neurolinguistic profile of Huntington's disease appears to differ from that Alzheimer's and Parkinson's (Illes 1989). Excessive loudness and pitch variations and vowel articulation abnormalities may also be present, partly due to iatrogenic effects of antipsychotic medication (Rusz et al. 2014). Understanding of discourse and semantic representation processing can also be subject to deterioration (Gagnon, Barrette and Macoir 2018). Systematic exploration of linguistic features of spontaneous narrative production in pre-symptomatic and early stage Huntington's disease indicates that numerous linguistic functions are declining along the disease progression and even before any abnormalities can be detected in other domains of neuropsychiatric testing. Fluency is affected in terms of unnecessary repetitions, truncations and anomalous pausing, while two other domains are markedly declining, namely, reference and connectivity. Difficulties in using determiners, grouping words into phrases, avoiding ambivalence, constructing grammatically correct complex sentences, implementing subordination of clauses, maintaining the flow of speech or setting the topic have been documented. Degeneration of putamen and other striatal structures as observed in concurrent imaging studies seems to correlate with mostly quantitative measures of linguistic production, such as the number of words per sentence (Hinzen et al. 2018).

As family members, patients and caretakers attest, a number of factors negatively impact communication in Huntington's disease, including emotional load, high pace in dialogues, insufficient eye contact, difficulty concentrating or personality changes. The loss or limitation of communication pathways is perceived as frustrating by both patients and family members (Hartelius et al. 2010). While communicating with Huntington patients, interlocutors should be aware of the necessity to adapt their own speech to particular needs of the patient, using shorter sentences and yes/no questions, eliminating unnecessary distractions, or implementing gestures as a supplemental means illustrating the meaning of spoken discourse. Due to increased latencies in understanding and speech production, a slower tempo may be necessary to facilitate dialogue (Hamilton et al. 2012). Spoken verbal communication in a subgroup of patients is further hampered by the presence of cortically and subcortically

conditioned auditory impairments that result in worsened speech processing
and sound source localization (Profant et al. 2017).

> *H., a juvenile Huntington's disease sufferer, was known to others*
> *as a smiling girl on a wheelchair, whose parents took the best care*
> *possible of her needs and invented an efficient system of alternative*
> *communication to learn the preferences of their daughter whenever*
> *possible. As H. did not exhibit marked chorea in her upper extremities*
> *and was able to precisely point her index finger to particular places*
> *despite being virtually incapable of speaking, the parents designed a*
> *printed alphabetical table tailored in size and readability to H.'s needs*
> *and carried it along on most occasions. The table could be easily put*
> *up on a wall or bulletin board with a sticker or an office magnet. With*
> *a charm of her own, H. was capable of pinpointing even long, complex*
> *words and sentences at the table until relatively advanced stages of*
> *disease.*
>   *(V., a sufferer's friend)*

Vignette 3.

Since social withdrawal and the status of being 'incommunicado'
contribute to the complex mesh of suffering experienced by patients,
maintaining the largest number of communication channels possible at
respective stages of Huntington's disease remains the main challenge for lay
caregivers and health professionals alike, including those that can directly
address the speaking and writing difficulties of the patient (a speech
language pathologist, an occupational therapist, a rehabilitation worker and
other members of the 'ideal' multidisciplinary team). While special
interventions and exercises, such as expiratory muscle strength training,
laryngeal relaxation techniques, articulation therapy, speech rhythm
exercises, or biofeedback, based on individual assessment, may help slow
down progression of the functional impairment of speech (Barkmeier-
Kraemer and Clark 2017), severe disability or complete loss of the ability to
speak usually follow in advanced disease. As fine motor skills and
intelligibility of speech deteriorate, it is often necessary to look for suitable

means of augmentative or alternative communication (Boss and Billie 2002).

Augmentative and alternative communication strategies in Huntington's disease may incorporate both low-tech and hi-tech instruments. No-tech (unaided) augmentative/alternative techniques, such as emphasized gestures or pantomime can sometimes be helpful to a limited extent. Unlike receptive capacity, productive capabilities can be facilitated or complemented in a number of ways by alphabet charts or pictorial (iconic/symbolic) tables and speech generating devices (also referred to as SGD's). Simple printed or hand-drawn display boards are appropriate for many basic purposes as long as adequate motor control is preserved, i.e., chorea or stiffness do not prevent the client from pointing their finger, hand or eye-gaze toward the picture representation of a letter or an object, property or action (notions usually embodied in nouns, adjectives and verbs, respectively). Eye-tracking input devices have also been designed for use in Huntington's disease, nevertheless, due to abnormalities in saccadic movements, they do not offer a viable communication opportunity for all sufferers (Blekher et al. 2006). Advanced functionality can be implemented in corresponding software tools in smartphones, tablets, laptops or desktops. Smartphones, however, may fail to provide enough space for motor-discoordinated users to be able to isolate the appropriate area of the communication grid displayed on the screen and may, therefore, be more suitable for simple yes/no applications (with screens divided into two large areas of different color pre-programmed as affirmative vs. dissenting answers). Perceived communicative involvement can be effectively enhanced by means of appropriate augmentative and alternative instruments, offering the patient a more intense feeling of socializing, interacting, belonging and comfort (Ferm et al. 2010; Fried-Oken, Mooney and Peters 2015).

Digital tools that enhance communication by Huntington patients and patients with other neurodegenerative diseases currently employ touchscreens of various sizes and/or specific types of voice-output generators as the most typical interfaces. If the motor status of the user, including involuntary movements, precludes adequately precise use of touchscreens and keyboards, indirect selection methods, such as various scanning input systems, can be utilized. A scanning input system allows the individual to select letters, words, pictures or phrases on the screen by controlling a simple combination of one or two switches. Typically, a box moves along the letter or picture arrays on an automatic or user-controlled basis until a click-selection is made. This procedure can be performed repeatedly until a desired word or combination of icons are formed (Elsahar et al. 2019). Although the communication rate is relatively slow, this type of input can be implemented even with grossly impaired motor skills and, thus, represents a beneficial expressive alternative for a subgroup of patients.

CONCLUSION

Naturally occurring emotions emerging as a reaction to distressing situations, such as disease and disability, as well as emotional disbalances assuming the shape of a defined psychiatric (mood, anxiety) disorder are a common occurrence in Huntington's disease patients. While the existing body of evidence indicates that numerous structural and functional biological abnormalities participate in this clinical picture, the most important aspect to be addressed with the limited means of treatment currently available is the subjective suffering of the patient and their family and functional disability caused by the disease process.

As the disease progresses, the patient's capacity to express themselves either verbally or non-verbally, ask for something, discuss various topics, verbalize preferences and socialize with relatives and friends becomes gradually more and more restricted. Such a limitation entails feelings of isolation, despair and frustration. Since advances in technology and rehabilitation offer an increasing number of modalities to apply in the amelioration of impaired communicative functions, it is imperative to involve both lay and professional caregivers, including speech language pathologists and biomedical technicians, as well as the patients themselves (to whatever extent their status permits) in the supplementation of deteriorating communication. Effective support of communication can attenuate the emotional impact of Huntington's disease on the patient.

Similarly, effective psychological support can keep Huntington patients motivated to engage in social interaction until more advanced treatment methods are available for this debilitating disease.

REFERENCES

Ahveninen, LM; Stout, JC; Georgiou-Karistianis, N; Lorenzetti, V; Glikmann-Johnston, Y. Reduced Amygdala Volumes Are Related to Motor and Cognitive Signs in Huntington's Disease: The IMAGE-HD Study. *NeuroImage. Clinical*, 18, (2018), 881-87. doi: 10.1016/j.nicl.2018.03.027.

Anderson, K; Eberly, S; Groves, M; Kayson, E; Marder, K; Young, AB; Shoulson, I. "Risk Factors for Suicidal Ideation in People at Risk for Huntington's Disease." *Journal of Huntington's Disease*, 5, no. 4, (2016), 389-94. doi: 10.3233/JHD-160206.

Barkmeier-Kraemer, JM; Clark, HM. "Speech-Language Pathology Evaluation and Management of Hyperkinetic Disorders Affecting Speech and Swallowing Function." *Tremor and Other Hyperkinetic Movements*, 7, (2017), 489. doi: 10.7916/D8Z32B30.

Bates, GP; Tabrizi, SJ; Jones, L. *Huntington's Disease*. Oxford: Oxford University Press, 2014.

Bindler, L; Touzeau, T; Travers, D; Millet, B. "Le Suicide Dans La Maladie De Huntington: état Actuel Des Connaissances." *Annales Médico-psychologiques, Revue Psychiatrique*, 168, no. 5, (2010), 338-42. doi:10.1016/j.amp.2009.12.017.

Blekher, TM; Johnson, SA; Marshall, JJ; White, KE; Hui, SCh; Weaver, M; Gray, JK; Yee, RM; Stout, JC; Beristain, X; Wojcieszek, JM; Foroud, T. "Saccades in Presymptomatic and Early Stages of Huntington Disease." *Neurology*, 67, no. 3, (2006), 394-99.

Bora, E; Velakoulis, D; Walterfang, M. Social Cognition in Huntington's Disease: A Meta-analysis. *Behavioral Brain Research*, 297, (2016), 131-40. doi: 10.1016/j.bbr.2015.10.001.

Boss, BJ; Billie, PR. "Communication: Language and Pragmatics." In *Rehabilitation Nursing: Process, Application & Outcomes*, 569-97, edited by S. P. Hoeman. St. Louis: Mosby, 2002.

Brandt, J. "Behavioral Changes in Huntington Disease." *Cognitive and Behavioral Neurology: Official Journal of the Society for Behavioral and Cognitive Neurology*, 31, no. 1, (2018), 26-35. doi: 10.1097/WNN. 0000000000000147.

Craufurd, D; Thompson, JC; Snowden, JS. "Behavioral Changes in Huntington Disease." *Neuropsychiatry, Neuropsychology and Behavioral Neurology*, 14, no. 4, (2001), 219-26.

Dale, M; van Duijn, E. "Anxiety in Huntington's Disease." *The Journal of Neuropsychiatry and Clinical Neurosciences*, 27, no. 4, (2015), 262-71. doi: 10.1176/appi.neuropsych.14100265.

Davis, M; Phillips, A; Tendler, A; Oberdeck, A. "Deep rTMS for Neuropsychiatric Symptoms of Huntington's Disease: Case Report." *Brain Stimulation*, 9, no. 6, (2016), 960-61. doi: 10.1016/j.brs.2016.09.002.

Durbach, N; Hayden, MR. "George Huntington: The Man behind the Eponym." *Journal of Medical Genetics*, 30, no. 5, (1993), 406-9. doi: 10.1136/jmg.30.5.406.

Ellis, D; Tucker, I. *Social Psychology of Emotion*. Los Angeles: SAGE, 2015.

Elsahar, Y; Hu, S; Bouazza-Marouf, K; Kerr, D; Mansor, A. "Augmentative and Alternative Communication (AAC) Advances: A Review of Configurations for Individuals with a Speech Disability." *Sensors*, 19, no. 8, (2019), 1911. doi: 10.3390/s19081911.

Epping, EA; Paulsen, JS. "Depression in the Early Stages of Huntington Disease." *Neurodegenerative Disease Management*, 1, no. 5, (2011), 407-14. doi: 10.2217/nmt.11.45.

Ferm, U; Sahlin, A; Sundin, L; Hartelius, L. "Using Talking Mats to support communication in persons with Huntington's Disease." *International Journal of Language & Communication*, 45, no. 5, (2010), 523-36. doi: 10.3109/13682820903222809.

Frankl, VE. *Man's Search for Meaning*. Boston: Beacon Press, 2006.

Frankl, VE. *On the Theory and Therapy of Mental Disorders. An Introduction to Logotherapy and Existential Analysis.* New York: Brunner-Routledge, 2004.

Fried-Oken, M; Mooney, A; Peters, B. "Supporting Communication for Patients with Neurodegenerative Disease." *NeuroRehabilitation*, 37, no. 1, (2015), 69-87. doi: 10.3233/NRE-151241.

Gagnon, M; Barrette, J; Macoir, J. "Language Disorders in Huntington Disease: A Systematic Literature Review." *Cognitive and Behavioral Neurology*, 31, no. 4, (2018), 179-92. doi: 10.1097/ WNN. 0000000000000171.¨

Hamilton, A; Ferm, U; Heemskerk, AW; Twiston-Davies, R; Matheson, K; Simpson, SA; Rae, D. "Management of Speech, Language and Communication Difficulties in Huntington's Disease." *Neurodegenerative Disease Management*, 2, no. 1, (2012), 67-77. doi: 10.2217/nmt.11.78.

Hartelius, L; Carlstedt, A; Ytterberg, M; Lillvik, M; Laakso, K. "Speech Disorders in Mild and Moderate Huntington Disease: Results of Dysarthria Assessments of 19 Individuals." *Journal of Medical Speech - Language Pathology*, 11, no. 1, (2003), 1-14.

Hartelius, L; Jonsson, M; Rickeberg, A; Laakso, K. "Communication and Huntington's Disease: Qualitative Interviews and Focus Groups with Persons with Huntington's Disease, Family Members, and Carers." *International Journal of Language and Communication Disorders*, 45, no. 3, (2010), 381-93. doi: 10.3109/13682820903105145.

Henley, SM; Novak, MJ; Frost, C; King, J; Tabrizi, SJ; Warren, JD. "Emotion Recognition in Huntington's Disease: A Systematic Review." *Neuroscience and Biobehavioral Reviews*, 36, no. 1, (2012), 237-53. doi: 10.1016/ j.neubiorev.2011.06.002.

Hinzen, W; Rosselló, J; Morey, C; Camara, E; Garcia-Gorro, C; Salvador, R; de Diego-Balaguer, R. "A Systematic Linguistic Profile of Spontaneous Narrative Speech in Pre-symptomatic and Early Stage Huntington's Disease." *Cortex*, 100, (2018), 71–83. doi:10.1016/ j.cortex.2017.07.022.

Ille, R; Holl, AK; Kapfhammer, HP; Reisinger, K; Schäfer, A; Schienle, A. "Emotion Recognition and Experience in Huntington's Disease: Is There a Differential Impairment?" *Psychiatry Research*, 188, no. 3, (2011), 377–82. doi: 10.1016/j.psychres.2011.04.007.

Illes, J. "Neurolinguistic Features of Spontaneous Language Production Dissociate Three Forms of Neurodegenerative Disease: Alzheimer's, Huntington's, and Parkinson's." *Brain and Language*, 37, no. 4, (1989), 628-42. doi: 10.1016/0093-934X(89)90116-8.

Kordsachia, CC; Labuschagne, I; Stout, JC. "Abnormal Visual Scanning of Emotionally Evocative Natural Scenes in Huntington's Disease." *Frontiers in Psychology*, 8, Article 405, (2017), 1-10. doi: 10.3389/fpsyg.2017.00405.

Kordsachia, CC; Labuschagne, I; Stout, JC. "Visual Scanning of the Eye Region of Human Faces Predicts Emotion Recognition Performance in Huntington's Disease." *Neuropsychology*, 32, no. 3, (2018), 356-65. doi: 10.1037/ neu0000424.

Kordsachia, CC; Labuschagne, I; Andrews, SC; Stout, JC. "Diminished Facial EMG Responses to Disgusting Scenes and Happy and Fearful Faces in Huntington's Disease." *Cortex*, 106, no. N/A, (2018), 185-99. doi: 10.1016/j.cortex.2018.05.019.

Krauss, R. The Psychology of Verbal Communication. In *International Encyclopedia of the Social & Behavioral Sciences*, edited by N. J. Smelser, and P. B. Baltes, 16161-65. New York: Elsevier, 2001.

Mason, SL; Zhang, J; Begeti, F; Guzman, NV; Lazar, AS; Rowe, JB; Barker, RA; Hampshire, A. "The Role of the Amygdala during Emotional Processing in Huntington's Disease: From Pre-manifest to Late Stage Disease." *Neuropsychologia*, 70, (2015), 80-89. doi: 10.1016/j.neuropsychologia.2015.02.017.

Mccolgan, P; Razi, A; Gregory, S; Seunarine, KK; Durr, A; Roos, RA; Leavitt, BR; Scahill, RI; Clark, CA; Langbehn, DR; Rees, G; Tabrizi, SJ. "Structural and Functional Brain Network Correlates of Depressive Symptoms in Premanifest Huntington's Disease." *Human Brain Mapping*, 38, no. 6, (2017), 2819-29. doi: 10.1002/hbm.23527.

Meiselman, HL. *Emotion Measurement*. Amsterdam: Elsevier, 2016.

Novak, MJ; Warren, JD; Henley, SM; Draganski, B; Frackowiak, RS; Tabrizi, SJ. "Altered Brain Mechanisms of Emotion Processing in Premanifest Huntington's Disease." *Brain*, 135, no. 4, (2012), 1165-79. doi: 10.1093/brain/aws024.

Osborne-Crowley, K; Andrews, SC; Labuschagne, I; Nair, A; Scahill, R; and Craufurd, D. "Apathy Associated With Impaired Recognition of Happy Facial Expressions in Huntington's Disease." *Journal of the International Neuropsychological Society*, 25, no. 5, (2019), 453-61. doi: 10.1017/ S1355617718001224.

Ossig, C; Storch, A. Depression in Huntington's disease. In *Neuropsychiatric symptoms of neurological disease. Neuropsychiatric symptoms of movement disorders, edited by* H. Reichmann, 201-9. Cham, Switzerland: Springer International Publishing, 2015.

Paoli, RA; Botturi, A; Ciammola, A; Silani, V; Prunas, C; Lucchiari, C; Caletti, E. "Neuropsychiatric Burden in Huntington's Disease." *Brain Sciences*, 7, no. 6, (2017): 67. doi: 10.3390/brainsci7060067.

Paulsen, JS; Ready, RE; Hamilton, JM; Mega, MS; Cummings, JL. "Neuropsychiatric Aspects of Huntington's Disease." *Journal of Neurology, Neurosurgery, and Psychiatry*, 71, no. 3, (2001), 310-14. doi: 10.1136/jnnp.71.3.310.

Phillips, JG; Bradshaw, JL; Chiu, E; Bradshaw, JA. "Characteristics of Handwriting of Patients with Huntington's Disease." *Movement Disorders*, 9, no. 5, (1994), 521-30. doi: 10.1002/mds.870090504.

Pla, P; Orvoen, S; Saudou, F; David, DJ; Humbert, S. "Mood Disorders in Huntington's Disease: From Behavior to Cellular and Molecular Mechanisms." *Frontiers in Behavioral Neuroscience*, 8, (2014), 135. doi: 10.3389/fnbeh.2014.00135.

Prochaska, JO; Norcross, JC. *Systems of Psychotherapy: A Transtheoretical Analysis*. Oxford: Oxford University Press, 2018.

Profant, O; Roth, J; Bureš, Z; Balogová, Z; Lišková, I; Betka, J; Syka, J. "Auditory Dysfunction in Patients with Huntington's Disease." *Clinical Neurophysiology*, 128, no. 10, (2017), 1946-53. doi:10.1016/ j.clinph.2017.07.403.

Quarrell, O. *Huntington's Disease: The Facts*. Oxford: Oxford University Press, 2008.

Pfaff, L; Lamy, J; Noblet, V; Gounot, D; Chanson, JB; De Seze, J; Blanc, F. "Emotional Disturbances in Multiple Sclerosis: A Neuropsychological and fMRI Study." *Cortex*, 117, (2019), 205-16. doi: 10.1016/j.cortex.2019.02.017.

Robotham, L; Sauter, DA; Bachoud-Lévi, AC; Trinkler, I. "The Impairment of Emotion Recognition in Huntington's Disease Extends to Positive Emotions." *Cortex*, 47, no. 7, (2011), 880-84. doi:10.1016/j.cortex.2011.02.014.

Rüb, U; Vonsattel, JPG; Heinsen, H; Korf, HW. *The Neuropathology of Huntington's Disease*. Cham: Springer International Publishing, 2015.

Rusz, J; Klempíř, J; Tykalová, T; Baborová, E; Cmejla, R; Růžička, E; Roth, J. "Characteristics and Occurrence of Speech Impairment in Huntington's Disease: Possible Influence of Antipsychotic Medication." *Journal of Neural Transmission*, 121, no. 12, (2014), 1529-39. doi: 10.1007/s00702-014-1229-8.

Schultz, JL; Killoran, A; Nopoulos, PC; Chabal, CC; Moser, DJ; Kamholz, JA. "Evaluating Depression and Suicidality in Tetrabenazine Users with Huntington Disease." *Neurology*, 91, no. 3, (2018). doi: 10.1212/wnl.0000000000005817.

Thompson, J; Harris, J; Sollom, AC; Stopford, C; Snowden, JS; Craufurd, D. "Longitudinal Evaluation of Neuropsychiatric Symptoms in Huntington's Disease." *The Journal of Neuropsychiatry and Clinical Neurosciences*, 24, no. 1, (2012), 53-60. doi: 10.1176/appi.neuropsych.11030057.

van Duijn, E. "Treatment of Irritability in Huntington's Disease." *Current Treatment Options in Neurology*, 12, no. 5, (2010), 424-33. doi: 10.1007/s11940-010-0088-3.

Reviewed by: J. Slonková, MD, PhD.

In: Living with Huntington's Disease ISBN: 978-1-53616-729-0
Editor: Sherman Howell © 2020 Nova Science Publishers, Inc.

Chapter 4

GENE THERAPY AS A POTENTIAL DECELERATOR OF THE HUNTINGTON'S DISEASE PROGRESSION

Cristiani Folharini Bortolatto[1,],*
Amália Gonçalves Alves[1], César Augusto Brüning[1],
Evelyn Mianes Besckow[1], Luiz Roberto Carraro Junior[1],
Jorge Mario Cárdenas Paredes[2,3], Rodolfo Baldinotti[1]
and Taís da Silva Teixeira Rech[1]

[1]Laboratory of Biochemistry and Molecular Neuropharmacology
(LABIONEM), Post-Graduate Program in Biochemistry and
Bioprospecting (PPGBBio), Center of Chemical,
Pharmaceutical and Food Sciences (CCQFA),
Federal University of Pelotas (UFPel)
[2]Laboratorio Genes SAS, Medellín, Colombia
[3]Grupo de Investigación en Genética Forense - Instituto Nacional de
Medicina Legal y Ciencias Forenses, Bogotá, Colombia

---

[*] Corresponding Author's E-mail: cbortolatto@gmail.com or cristiani.bortolatto@ufpel.edu.br.

ABSTRACT

Huntington's disease (HD) is a genitive inheritance pathology disease that causes pleiotropic symptoms, including motor, cognitive, and psychiatric impairments. Mutations in the HTT gene (Ch.4 p. 16.3) cause the expansion of the CAG trinucleotide repeat region of the HTT gene, generating a long abnormal version of the huntingtin (HTT) protein. Moreover, the cell machinery forms small protein aggregates that accumulate in neurons, disrupting the normal cell functions. Current HD clinical treatments focus on attenuating symptoms with conventional therapies and pharmacological treatments, with limited effectiveness. Under those circumstances, current research aims to find new targets to promote the reduction of HD severity in patients. Recent evidence suggests that several neural functions regulated by epigenetic imprinting are disrupted in HD patients, resulting in the typical portrait of HD neuronal disorders. For instance, clinical and pre-clinical data of the epigenetic processes in HD indicate alterations in its regulatory pathways. In fact, epigenetic abnormalities namely, DNA methylation, post-translational modifications in nucleosome histones and biogenesis of the miRNA are dysregulated in HD´s experimental models and HD patients. Moreover, recent developments silencing HTT RNA messenger molecules through Antisense Oligonucleotides and its posterior degradation via RNase H1 enzyme have shown a significant reduction on mutant HTT protein expression in HD patients. These findings and recent research advances have set new research horizons to therapeutic targets and the establishment of more effective clinical treatments. Therefore, this chapter describes current trends and efforts in gene therapy techniques, and the improvements in health conditions of HD patients and their families.

Keywords: Huntington Disease, Mutant Huntingtin, epigenetic abnormalities, gene therapy

INTRODUCTION

According to Brazil's Huntington Association, the Huntington Disease (HD) is a genetic and progressive inheritance pathology that affects the central nervous system (CNS). Nowadays, there is no effective treatment or definitive cure for HD patients; however, in most of the cases, patients experience normal life for several years before the onset of symptoms. HD is mainly caused by an abnormal expansion of polyglutamine (polyQ) amino acid residues in the gene coding the huntingtin (HTT) protein [1]. Even though there is no definitive treatment for HD, as happens with other genetic diseases, research has relied on gene therapy [2], with the aim to manipulate nucleic acids to replace or correct defective genes or gene products to support the cell, improving the disease treatment [3].

By the 1960s, human therapy was first considered and was mainly directed with the idea of transferring genes to the human genome using viruses [4], but it was not until the next decade that Paul Berg began to manipulate deoxyribonucleic acid (DNA) molecules developing new techniques and resulting in what we nowadays know as recombinant DNA technology [5]. Gene therapy attempts failed to succeed during the preceded years until 1989 when a new method raised positive perspectives to the field. The method was tested in a clinical trial with a four-year-old patient that was not capable of expressing adenosine deaminase (ADA) enzyme, resulting in T-cells adulteration in the immune system [6]. During a period between one and two months, researchers extracted T cells from the patient's blood and introduced the ADA enzyme gene inducing its proliferation in cell culture and later reintroduced them back in her bloodstream [7]. According to method mentioned above, the trial was done and six-month breaks were given until the treatment completed two years. In the end, this was the first case where gene therapy gave positive results because ADA levels increased and remained stable along with the six-month break [8, 9]. By 2010, after twelve years of this therapy, the treatment already showed that T-cells on the patient bloodstream remained expressing the therapeutic gene [10].

The concept of gene therapy consists of the introduction of genes in the cell. However, the natural entrance of the exogenous DNA through the membrane of eukaryotic cells is extremely rare and restricted by cell mechanisms. Therefore, a biological carrier would be always needed to simplify the entrance of exogenous DNA in the living cells and are generally known as vectors. There are three main types of vectors used in biotechnology: viral vectors, plasmids and nanostructured vectors [11, 12]. In general, clinical trials have been demonstrated that viral vectors are more efficient at gene delivery *in vivo* than synthetic nanoparticle and plasmids. [13].

Viral vectors rely on the biology of viruses, which are specialized agents in invading and introducing its genetic material (DNA or RNA) to the host cell nucleus [11]. Generally, viruses have two ways to replicate their genetic material. One of them is to invade the cell and use the cell's replication machinery to replicate itself and lysing the host cell in the process (lytic cycle). The second is to integrate its genome into the host genome and replicate every time the host cell undergoes cell division in a non-pathogenic fashion (lysogenic cycle). The latter is known to be done by the retroviruses and lentiviruses, which are the most used viral vectors for gene therapy [13].

Furthermore, molecular and gene-based therapies are now the emerging therapeutic approaches for HD studies, with the aim of slowing down or even reducing to the minimum the inherent health risks. In this context, several gene/molecular interventions are now under development for HD [14]. Researchers are focusing their attention and efforts on reducing the mutated HTT (mHTT) mRNA levels and up to date, the most efficient methods are the ones built to overcome the transcript using short hairpin RNAs (shRNAs) and artificial microRNAs (miRNAs) scaffolds. Data show that reduction of HTT in murine HD models using adeno-associated viral (AAV) vectors is significant and methods using shRNA or miRNA provide a long-term silencing of the HTT transcript, avoiding a re-administration therapy [15].

Besides, HD patients are unable to regulate correctly the DNA methylation patterns of their genes compromising cell identity [16]. The methylation pattern of the cell is done by the DNA methyltransferase (DNMT), an enzyme responsible for methylating DNA over the gene's CpG (cytosine-guanine) islands. Although DNA methylation is the most analyzed epigenetic mechanism for many diseases, applications on HD therapy are still on their initial stages [17].

Another feature found in HD is that patients are more prone to develop a defective neuronal histone acetylation pattern [18]. Histone acetylation patterns are epigenetic marks that regulate expression of genes using the histone-DNA interactions by the histone deacetylases (HDACs) and histone acetyltransferases (HATS) enzymes. Data show that acetylation patterns in HD become abnormal due to an anomalous deacetylation activity done by HDACs enzymes. This results in a shutdown of gene expression and condensation of chromatin disabling the correct gene transcription [19].

Advances in molecular approaches for HD therapy development are translating into the design of non-traditional clinical trials for HD. Related to those approaches, a recent study has evaluated the willingness of potential participants in different trials of HD molecular therapy through an anonymous survey distributed through the Huntington's Disease Society of America (HDSA) portal. The authors revealed that the HD population has a high willingness to participate in gene therapy trials [14]. Also, in addition to ongoing clinical trials of Roche/Genentech and Wave HTT-lowering therapies, a number of other companies are developing drugs aiming at lowering levels of mHTT in the body and brain. These novel approaches rely on "gene therapy" has the potential to treat diseases [20]. One important example is the candidate AMT-130, a gene therapy product developed by uniQure aiming at inhibiting the production of the mHTT, which received U.S. Food and Drug Administration (FDA) fast track designation [21].

It is important to say that gene therapy has ethical and public policy questions that still being part of discussions around the community. In the past, the response to this technique was ethical unease and even fear of some human administrations of molecular genetics in the philosophical, scientific, religious, theological and public policy societies and even among some calm advocacy groups. However, a constructive optimism prevailed and it was resolved quickly through public discussion and clarification of the ethical varieties between germline genetic modification and somatic gene therapy [22, 23].

MECHANISMS OF HD

Effective gene therapy relies on the identification of pathways and the physio-pathological alterations caused by the disease. As mentioned above, the core of the different forms of disease manifestion is mainly associated with the mutated version of the HTT gene. Mutations in the HTT gene (Ch.4 p. 16.3) causes an aberrant expansion of the CAG trinucleotide repeat region in the exon 1 of the gene, generating a long abnormal version of the HTT protein, characterized by an expanded polyglutamine domain. The protein HTT is ubiquitously expressed in all tissues, but its function is not totally understood. Researchers believe that it is involved in various cellular processes, namely on gene transcription, apoptosis and intracellular transport. In HD patients, the mHTT acquires a toxic feature for the cell. It is currently recognized that neurodegeneration is caused not only by the toxic effect of mHTT but also by the loss of wild-type HTT [1, 24].

Other neurodegenerative diseases are also characterized by a protein dysfunction, occurring difficulty in eliminating inefficient proteins, which leads to the formation of intracellular aggregates. The mHTT is subject of proteolytic cleavage, producing fragments that tend to form aggregates which are situated in the nucleus and in the cytoplasm. mHTT fragments can induce the opening of the mitochondrial permeability transition pore, resulting in the release of cytochrome C. Once in the cytosol, cytochrome C mediates the activation of caspases, which, in turn, can cleave the mHTT and promotes its translocation into the nucleus [1]. Mitochondrial dysfunction in HD has been well documented with the progression of the disease and is found in different tissues including brain, skeletal muscle, and heart. Also, it is observed an increased accumulation of damaged mitochondria in the lysosome that has been coupled with lysosomal dysfunction [25].

Other mechanisms quite affected by HD are the synaptic plasticity and neurotransmitter release. The most affected region in the brain with HD is the striatum, a relatively small structure, located under the cortex. Over the course of HD, the striatum and cortex tend to shrink and eventually cause tissue damage [26]. Striatal projection neurons (SPNs) are not equally vulnerable to the disease, and data show that HD patient's brain exhibit alterations even before the SPNs start degenerating. The changes in neural activity observed in HD are related to an abnormal and interconnected release of neurotransmitters [27]. Because mHTT is responsible for alterations on synaptic transmission, some neurotransmitters implicated in these processes will be discussed below.

Dopamine plays an important role in muscular movement, behavior, motivation and reward. Dopamine release is notably reduced because of the progression of HD's phenotype. Chorea, a characteristic symptom of HD patients related with involuntary movements, seems to be the result of impairment and alteration in the excitation pattern of dopamine receptors which later decrease making the distinctive features displayed in HD patients. Therefore, a dopamine stabilization is fundamental for the treatment of HD patients [1, 28, 29].

Besides dopamine, glutamate (a stimulating neurotransmitter of SPNs) is also related to the neurodegenerative process of the disease. Glutamate release and uptake dysregulation may stimulate defective synaptic reorganization and loss of synapses [29]. N-methyl-d-aspartate (NMDA) receptors found in SPNs, are ionotropic glutamatergic receptor composed of two subunits: GluN1 and a combination of two GluN2 (A and B). Normally, GluN2B subunits are highly expressed in SPNs; however, mHTT enhances the expression of these subunits in the surface, being almost wholly extra-synaptic. In this sense, mHTT causes enhanced NMDA sensitivity and alteration of NMDAR expression and localization in neurons. Damage caused by glutamatergic disturbances in these communication mechanisms may be higher than the cellular pathways of surviving and plasticity. In fact, the overstimulation of NMDA receptors activates pathways that result in excitotoxicity and promote stress and cellular death. Among the NMDAR subunits involved in glutamatergic-mediated excitotoxicity, the GluN2B subunit receptor has been extensively reported [30, 31].

It is notable that both excitatory and inhibitory signals affect the motor and cognitive functions of HD patients. Inhibitory interneurons are also involved with movements, so the loss of these synapses would lead to the involuntary movement characteristic of chorea. GABAergic interneurons represent about 5% of neurons of striatum corpus and reports indicate that GABA-related circuits are compromised in the pathogenesis of HD. Therefore, mHTT is responsible for the alteration in the GABA release and consequently, a malfunctioning inhibitory system could be unable to suppress the involuntary movements [32, 33]. The disruption of synaptic function and plasticity in HD affects a variety of synaptic signaling molecules on various neuronal types and brain structures. The neurotransmitters above mentioned are notoriously studied for the characterization of their involvement in HD, since some changes in signaling, such as reduced transcription and transport, are a direct result of the effect of mHTT. Therefore, alteration of wild-type HTT activity and neuron synapses, are typical HD symptoms, leading to neuronal instability and cell death [34].

In addition to the protein aggregation, neurotransmitters dysfunction, and aberrant neural synapses, mHTT is also related to mitochondrial dysfunction, resulting in neurodegenerative processes [35]. Even before HTT protein aggregates appear, mitochondrial dysfunction may be responsible for early symptoms in HD [36]. Research indicates that mitochondrial dysfunction may increase the concentration of lactate in the striatum complex and cerebrospinal fluid. As a consequence, impairments of ATP formation and deregulation of glucose uptake occur in these regions [1, 37, 38, 39]. Mitochondria are responsible for apoptosis pathways, regulating intracellular levels of calcium ions and reactive oxygen species (ROS) needed to activation of apoptotic enzymes. Studies have pointed out an evident and significant increase in ROS content in HD patients, consistent with the HD pathogenesis. Oxidative stress is also one of the early features reported in HD, but it is not already known whether it is a consequence of mitochondrial dysregulation itself or is a direct consequence of mHTT [41, 49].

As described above, mHTT promotes changes mainly in the striatum complex; however, because it is ubiquitously expressed, its impacts are likewise present in various neuronal and glial cells. Astrocytes, the most abundant glial cells in the brain, are associated with the metabolic support to neurons and synaptic transmission, and they are equally affected by mHTT [42]. Reports in transgenic mice expressing N-terminal mHTT in astrocytes display weight loss changes and motor function impairments with notable shorter lifespan compared with wild-type and controls, consistent with the disease physiopathology. As a result, HD disease seems to affect the glial cells and dysregulate the expression of miRNA and glutamatergic transporter pathways, causing the non-removal of glutamate from the synaptic cleft and the typical excitotoxicity portrait [43].

As described, there are several therapy targets to deal with the HD, although deeper research and multifactorial analyses are necessary to be done because of the complexity of the disease. So, therapy design may not only consider assessing a unique target, but others may be taken into account. Since above-mentioned dysregulations are closely related (protein aggregation, mitochondrial dysfunction, synapses, and neurotransmitters release) many therapeutic approaches are primarily focused on the modification of mHTT, a topic that will be discussed later in this chapter.

GENE EXPRESSION REGULATION BY MICRORNAS

The miRNAs are small non-coding RNA molecules (20 to 25 nucleotides long) that play an important role in gene expression. miRNAs link to the 3'-UTR of mRNA targets and recruit the silencer complex induced by RNA (RISC) to inhibit the target expression [44, 45]. The RNA polymerase II will transcribe the miRNA primary genes (pri-miRNA), thus producing an incomplete stem-loop structure several thousand bases long [46]. The pri-miRNA will be processed by the microprocessor complex (cleaved by DROSHA) in the nucleus and may generate precursor miRNA (pre-miRNAs) which present a 70 nucleotides structure. After the nucleus exportation by exportina 5, the pre-miRNAS are usually cleaved by Dicer to generate mature miRNAs [45, 47]. The miRNAs are conserved in various animal species, showing a deep effect on gene expression, indicating the evolution and highlighting the role of these molecules as modulators of many biological pathways and processes, like metabolism control, cell cycle, cell differentiation, among other factors. In some pathologies, a higher or lower expression of miRNA's levels have been observed. Based on that, investigating these small molecules enables their use as candidates to a new class of drugs, the "miRNA therapeutics" [48].

Perspectives of miRNAs as Therapeutic Agents for HD

The miRNA therapy can be divided into three categories: mimetic miRNAs, miRNA inhibitors (also known as antimiRs), and antagomiRs. Mimetic miRNAs are small RNA molecules that combine with the constitutive miRNA and reinforce the expression of miRNAs who have lost their normal activity due to the disease, while antimiRs are based on antisense oligonucleotides, which can hybridize the miRNA and block the translation into protein. Basically, antagomiRs are small synthetic RNA molecules presenting a complementary sequence to the inhibited miRNA, which block the function of given miRNA, strongly bonding to each other. Several challenges in the usage of these techniques are still studied and searches for solutions are still being held. One example is the degradation of oligonucleotides by RNAs in the serum. Strategies for the application of these miRNAs are much explored such as chemical alterations in oligonucleotides, methylation of nucleotides, locked nucleic acids, among others. The addition of phosphorothioate groups and development of carrier vehicles (nanoparticles) promote the delivery of miRNA, thus keeping the molecule stability and avoiding its degradation [48].

Therapies using miRNAs have increased, not only directed to HD but also to other pathologies. The miRNAs show the complexity and enable us to understand a bit about human biology. Studies for the identification of miRNAs involved in HD are of extreme relevance. From this, it is possible to select the miRNAs involved in the disease and thus generate targeted therapy. Through current techniques of sequencing along with the use of human samples, the identification of the expression of a set of miRNAs misregulated with the progression of the disease was possible. In the Brodman area 4 (BA4), where miR-218, miR-196a, and miR- 486, are highly expressed in the pathological region, miR-132, miR-9, miR-124a, miR-29b, and miR-22, have low expression in patients with HD [49]. It also found that miR-100, miR-15, miR-151-3p, miR-219-2-3p, miR-451, miR-27b and miR-92a were over-regulated in the striatum and frontal cortex of HD patients, while miR-128, miR-222, miR-139-3p, miR-382, miR-483-3p, and miR-433 were repressed in diseased tissues [49].

In healthy neurons, transcriptional repressor RE1-Silencing Transcription factor (REST) is expressed at low levels and sequestered in the cytoplasm through interaction with HTT, but in patients with HD, the mHTT cannot bind to REST and is translocated to the nucleus [50]. In the nucleus, it can recruit corepressors (CoREST) and methyl-binding protein CpG 2 (MeCP2) causing inactivation of neuron-specific genes [50, 51, 52]. Thus, REST controls the expression of miRNAs presenting indirect consequences in the deregulation of the HD gene expression [49]. This repressor leads to an increase in transcriptional repression of brain-derived neuronal factor (BDNF) which is related to neuronal survival and neurogenesis. The BDNF downregulation in the striatum of HD patients contributes to the clinical manifestations of the disease [53].

miR9 / miR-9 *, a miRNA regulated by REST, targets two components of the REST silencing complex. Total RNA has been isolated to analyze miRNAs that are affected with HD progression. It was found that five REST-regulated miRNAs were significantly reduced with increasing HD grade, miR-9 / miR-9 *, miR-29b, miR-124a and miR-132 [54]. REST has an interaction with CoREST and other transcriptional repressors to regulate neuronal gene expression through its direct control of mRNA and also with miRNA transcripts [52, 55, 56, 57]. Many *in vitro* studies have shown that the forced expression of miRNA-124 in some non-neuronal cells promotes neuronal differentiation. In addition, excessive expression of miR-124 in non-neuronal cells induces gene expression profiles to a neuronal phenotype [58].

A recent study shows that miRNA-124 is a determinant of neuronal fate in the subventricular zone, in which inhibition *in vivo* of miRNA-124 blocked neurogenesis in that region since its expression is related to neuroplasticity and differentiation [59]. Interestingly, genes related to neurogenesis are highly represented among altered genes in the expression in the cortex (BA4) of HD patients [60]. Remarkably, REST proteins from the cell lysate were upregulated in mice via miRNA-124 injection, but it is unknown if the increased REST proteins were from the nucleus or cytoplasm. Therefore, it was not possible to determine whether REST has repressed activation. However, the target of REST, BDNF, was increased by the injection of miRNA-124 implying that increased REST did not cause translocation to the nucleus to repress transcription. Low BDNF levels are detected in patients with HD and mouse models, and the loss of BDNF in the brain leads to more neuronal loss [61, 62, 63, 64, 65]. In the same study, microRNA-124 markedly increased levels of PGC-1α protein and BDNF, suggesting a protective function in neuronal survival. MicroRNA-124 has shown positive effects by slowing the progression of HD, promoting neurogenesis in the striatum and improving neuronal survival. Collectively, miRNA-124 is a promising therapeutic strategy for HD [65].

Additionally, miRNA-132 has been reported to target methyl CpG-binding protein 2 (MeCP2), a known regulator of neural maturation. It has been reported that the loss of MeCP2 decreased the levels of BDNF by REST/CoRest-mediated repression [66, 67, 68]. The miRNA-132 is strongly associated with neuronal maturation. Experiments with miRNA-132 showed an improvement in HD symptoms and interferences in disease progression in animal models, so it can be a therapeutic method for alleviating symptoms and delaying the HD progression in humans [69].

miR-132 supplemental treatment to the brain caused a reduction of symptoms of disease in R6/2 mice (HD model), despite of a little effect on disease-causing mHTT mRNA expression and its products in the striatum, a major HD focus. In addition, a miR-132 reduction has been found in both striata of R6/2 mice and brains of HD patients assessed by *postmortem* techniques [70], reinforcing the association between miR-132 and HD. The AAV9_miR-132 virus appears to provide sufficient miR-132 to compensate for a miR-132 deficiency in the HD brain. The miRNA-132 therapy can become adjuvant by delaying the onset and progression of the disease; however, the miRNA-132 enhancing mechanism in the brain has not yet been elucidated [69].

Deregulation of miRNA-22 expression has been implicated in the pathogenesis of various neurodegenerative diseases [53]. The increase in cellular miRNA-22 levels may be an approach to combat neurodegeneration. The overexpression of miR-22 has been shown to be neuroprotective *in vitro* models of HD. It is explained by the relationship between the HD pathogenesis and abnormalities related with Rcor1, hypoacetylation of histone HDAC4 and regulator of G-protein signaling 2 (Rgs2) [53, 70]. Recent findings have demonstrated that inhibition of Rgs2 is protective in HD. The mechanisms underlying the effects of miR-22 include a reduction in caspase activation, consistent with miR-22's, targeting the pro-apoptotic activities of mitogen-activated protein kinase 14/p38 (MAPK14/p38) and tumor protein p53-inducible nuclear protein 1 (Tp53inp1). These properties stimulate the research to use miRNA-22 for therapeutic purposes, not only for HD but for other neurodegenerative pathologies [70].

Viral Vectors as miRNA Carriers

Currently, studies using viruses as vectors to lead transfer and express genetic material to target cells are being done, and have been showing positive results for the management of neurodegenerative diseases, although complementary studies are needed to use this technique, in order to increase the efficiency of this method, and safety for patients using it [71]. Among the vectors that can be used are lentiviruses, adenoviruses, and adeno-associated virus (AAV) [72]. These vectors can be differentiated in some aspects, such as how they deliver genetic material, whether they have a viral factor or not, and how they construct modification of genetic material in the target cell [73]. Different techniques with the use of viruses in gene therapy include the use of non-viral vectors, which are composed of synthetically produced biological particles. The DNA plasmid containing the therapeutic transgene is encapsulated with a chemical compound or RNA fragments. In order to build those biological particles, the genes for virus pathogenicity are removed, and the genes of interest are inserted. The adeno-associated virus (AAV) genome contains a single strand which consists of three genes, Rep (Replication), Cap (Capsid), and aap (Assembly). Recombinant AAV (rAAV), which has no viral DNA, is a protein-based nanoparticle designed to cross the cell membrane, where it can finally travel and deliver its DNA charge to the nucleus of a cell [73, 74, 75, 76].

The use of AAV has the advantage of crossing the blood-brain barrier, which is not possible with large molecules, and also allows the transduction directly into the target cells, for example, astrocytes. As mentioned earlier, astrocytes as well as neuronal cells suffer impairment of HD function and can cause astrogliosis [73]. In the case of GLT1, a glutamatergic astrocyte transporter that is deficient in transgenic HD carriers, the use of AAV appeared to improve the cellular conditions of those cells. AAV is characterized by low immunogenicity, ability to transduce cells in the division phase or not, broad cell tropism and the use of non-pathogenic host viruses. However, it is possible that an immune response of the organism will occur and still result in different transductions depending on the body profile in which the therapy is inserted [77].

HD-directed therapies aim to provide miRNA using recombinant AAV (rAAV) systems. Several experiments with animal models (R6/2 mice) have been conducted, showing positive effects, as symptom reduction and slowing the progression of the disease. It is important to note that the miRNA-based approach to AAV release gene therapy comprises the continuous expression of artificial miRNAs after a single administration of an AAV vector [26]. Another use of AAV is related to the changes that mHTT promotes in the skeletal muscles, leading to a decrease in the body weight of patients with the disease, a characteristic clinical condition of HD. Furthermore, the use of a virus-specific serotype, AAV9, reduced the expression of mutated proteins in transgenic animals. Specifically, this AAV serotype is able to transduce neuronal and glial cells not only in the brain but also in peripheral tissues, seeking to reduce expressed mHTT and also prevent disease-induced lesions [41].

APPLICATION OF EPIGENETIC MODELS IN HD

There has been increasing interest in the roles of epigenetic factors in the pathological mechanisms of HD, considering that through these mechanisms new possible therapies can be elaborated. These epigenetic factors include histone modifications and DNA methylation [78], which are associated with transcriptional rupture leading to the disease phenotypes. Environmental factors also cause epigenetic changes that may alter gene expression, such as DNA methylation. It is not yet clear exactly how mHTT protein leads to neuronal degeneration and neuropathological manifestations [79].

General Characteristics of DNA Methylation

DNA methylation is one of the most studied epigenetic modifications in mammals and is a critical agent in the proper regulation of gene expression and gene silencing [80]. This modification involves the covalent addition of a methyl group at the 5-position on the cytosine pyrimidine ring, creating 5-methylcytosine (5-mC) and reaches the human genome covering 4-6% of all cytosines and 60-80% of all the dinucleotide CpG [81]. The functions of DNA methylation are mediated in part by a family of DNA binding proteins. Mutations in MeCP2, a CpG methylation reader highly expressed in mature neurons, leading to deficits in neural development and neuronal functions. They are linked to syndromes that cause severe neurodevelopmental disorder in humans [82].

The discovery of 5-hydroxymethylcytosine (5hmC), an oxidation product of 5mC and potential epigenetic modifier, has broadened the range of effects in neurodegenerative diseases. Five DNMTs were identified in mammals catalyzes the cytosine methylation reaction: DNMT1, DNMT2, DNMT3a, DNMT3b, and DNMT3L are expressed throughout neural development and promote neuronal survival and plasticity [83]. The DNMT is classified in *de novo* methylation DNMTs (DNMT3a e DNMT3b) and DNMTs of maintenance (DNMT1). The DNMT3a and DNMT3b can establish a new pattern of methylation in the non-modified DNA. The DNMTs of maintenance act during the replication of DNA to copy the methylation pattern of the parental DNA strand to the newly synthesized strand. Therefore, only three members of the DNMT family directly catalyze the addition of methyl groups on the DNA: DNMT1, DNMT3a and DNMT3b [84].

DNMT1 is the enzyme related to maintenance of methylations, gene regulation, and chromatin stability. Studies suggest that mutations in

DNMT1 cause hereditary neurodegeneration [85]. Methylation of cytosines in CpG dinucleotides is often associated with the repression of specific gene expression since it generally interferes with the binding of transcription factors. It may also be involved in the interaction with the methyl-CpG binding proteins [86, 87]. Altered DNA methylation was found in patients with HD and in tests with transgenic mice with HD. Those studies have demonstrated that the Sox2, Pax6, and Nes genes are highly methylated, and the expression levels of these genes are significantly reduced in HD patients. These genes are directly involved in neurogenesis and may be related to symptoms, including cognitive decline [88, 89].

The relation between the mHTT expression and altered methylations that cause DNA transformation was reported through HD autopsies [90]. These mutations may alter the regulation of chromatin during neuronal development thus contributing to symptoms of HD [91]. Studies with human fibroblasts obtained from HD patients demonstrated changes in 5-mC [92]. Another type of mutation related to HD is transcription alterations in adenosine A_{2A} receptors that are abundant in spiny neurons. However, in people with HD, there is a decrease in these receptors, making this neuronal subtype more vulnerable and this mechanism a possible therapeutic target [93, 94]. Other studies have demonstrated the link between the reduction of adenosine A_{2A} receptors with the high level of 5-mC in patients affected with HD, demonstrating a relationship with the epigenetic regulation which reinforces the idea that DNA methylation may be a relevant factor for the pathogenesis of HD [94, 95, 96, 97].

In addition to the methylation of 5-cytosine, there are other types of methylation less studied, such as guanine methylation, which has been shown to be related to the pathology of HD. According to studies conducted by Thomas and collaborators, 7-methylguanosine (7-mG) levels were found to be significantly altered in the brain models of animals affected with HD compared with the control groups [98]. Through this, DNA methylation is suggested being one of the epigenetic alterations that contribute to the pathogenesis of HD. However, there are many questions still to be studied, such as the way the HTT mutation triggers DNA methylation. Another question is how DNMTs and factors of DNA methylation maintenance are involved in epigenetic modifications in HD. In addition, preclinical studies with animals have demonstrated that inhibition of histone deacetylase (HDAC) may cause changes in DNA methylation leading to phenotypes that are milder in HD [92].

Histone Modifications

Acetylation and methylation are the most studied genomic modifications that affect the association of histone proteins with DNA. These histone modifications affect the chromatin fibers that consequently interfere in this interaction [78]. Histones are central components of the nucleosome subunits and are involved in gene expression. Gene expression is regulated by two components that act together: the binding of transcriptional activators and repressors, and the alteration of chromatin structure controlled by histone modification and chromatin remodeling [99]. Histone tails have a (N)-terminal amino acid moiety which is strongly basic and contain specific amino acid residues, which may result in susceptible post-translational covalent modifications (PTMs) including methylation and acetylation. It is known that histones directly affect the plasticity of chromatin structure, so these modifications can affect processes such as transcription, mitosis and impair chromosomal stability [100]. In general, acetylation of amino acid residues corresponds to transcriptionally active chromatin, while methylation leads to transcriptional repression. Many combinations of covalent modifications are possible on the central histones.

Histone modification patterns appear to be the key factor in the activation or deactivation of specific genes. The transfer of acetyl-Coa to NH_3 molecules coupled to an amino acid residue orchestrates the acetylation and deacetylation process. These residues linked to histone tails decrease the electrostatic interactions between histones and DNA [101]. Histone acetylation and deacetylation are modulated by the interaction between HATs and HDACs, widely studied as a possible therapeutic target. They act on repair to modify the structure of chromatin and regulate transcription [99].

Histone Acetylation in HD

Impairments in transcriptional activation and repression regulated by chromatin acetylation have been found in HD pathology [101]. Histone acetyl-transferases and histone deacetylases (HDACs) are responsible for performing the acetylation and deacetylation of histone proteins, respectively [19]. It is now becoming increasingly clear that several neurodevelopmental, neurodegenerative, and neuropsychiatric disorders are caused by aberrant changes in chromatin acetylation [102]. Histones are hypoacetylated in mouse models of HD, and there are strong indications that histone deacetylase inhibitors might be of therapeutic benefit in this condition [99].

Additionally, the reinstating acetylation homeostasis has been suggested as ameliorative condition mediated by the action of a histone acetylase (HAT) modulator for neurodegenerative disorders [102]. The striatal kinase DCLK3 has been showed to produce neuroprotection against mHTT by playing a key role in transcription regulation and chromatin remodeling in brain cells; the kinase domain seems to interact with zinc finger proteins, including the transcriptional activator adaptor TADA3, a core component of the Spt-ada-Gcn5 acetyltransferase (SAGA) complex which links histone acetylation to the transcription machinery [103]. Furthermore, histone deacetylases contribute differently to HTT polyglutamine toxicity in *Caenorhabditis elegans* [104], and histone deacetylase 6 inhibition has been related to the compensation of the transport deficit in HD [105].

Research has also shown that the acetylation of histones is reduced in cells expressing mutant polyglutamine. This suggests that the nuclear accumulation of polyglutamine may lead to the alteration of protein acetylation in neurons and indicate a new therapeutic strategy for polyglutamine diseases such as HD [106, 107]. Genetic research on polyglutamine diseases indicates that mutant proteins containing polyglutamine expansions assume toxic properties involved in the etiology of disease [108]. Perutz and collaborators proposed that expanded polyglutamine tracts could alter the solubility and folding properties of the proteins in which they were inserted. *In vitro* experiments have demonstrated that polyglutamine tracts can form insoluble aggregates with amyloid fibril-like properties [109]. The exact mechanism of how homeostasis is affected by the reduction of acetylation is not yet fully elucidated, but recent studies showed a link with the transcriptional dysfunction [110].

Histone Methylation in HD

Post-translational modification of histones by methylation is an important and widespread process which affects the regulation of gene transcription and is known by influencing biological processes in the context of development and cellular responses. The methylation/demethylation modifications can occur in all basic amino acid residues such as arginines, lysines, and histidines [111] and involve one, two, or three methyl groups. Histone methylation occurs predominantly on histones H3 and H4, and it is noteworthy that those alterations in histone methylation status have been linked to a large number of human diseases [112].

A role for FAD-dependent lysine-specific demethylase (KDM1) in brain function has emerged offering additional opportunities for the development of novel therapeutic strategies in neurodegenerative disease [112]. In addition, Song and colleagues [113] carried out systematic genetic interaction studies, testing lysine and arginine methylases and demethylases in a *Drosophila melanogaster* HD model and identified histone demethylase Utx as a potential target for ameliorating HD. Furthermore, the protein level of trimethylated histone H3K9 and ESET gene expression were elevated in HD patients and in R6/2 mice as demonstrated by the study conducted by Ryu and co-workers [114], and the alterations were attenuated by combined pharmacological treatment with mithramycin and cystamine. A lower level of histone H3 Lys4 (K4) (H3K4) methylation was found in the brains of first filial generation (F1) offspring from HD transgenic mice treated with an HDAC1/3-targeting inhibitor. This finding was related with improved HD disease phenotypes [92].

One of the most important arginine methylations can be found in H4 histones given that it is an important target for methylation and is associated with transcriptional activation [101]. Several types of arginine methyltransferases (PRMTs) perform methylation modifications of arginine, and studies have shown that mHTT protein has a PRMT5 deficiency and this fact may be associated with the pathogenesis of HD [115].

CLINICAL STUDIES BASED ON HD

Overview

Dysfunction of epigenetic components and alteration of epigenetic modifications have been closely linked to the pathogenesis of HD, as shown by some results with HDAC inhibitors in preclinical trials. A broad spectrum of HDAC inhibitors such as sodium butyrate (NaB), suberoylanilide hydroxamic acid (SAHA) and trichostatin A (TSA) has been used in clinical trials to demonstrate the relationship between the HDAC inhibition and the defective neuronal histone acetylation with abnormalities generated by HD [92]. Studies using sodium phenylbutyrate as an HDAC inhibitor have reported an increase in the miRNA in the blood of patients with HD, indicating positive effects as improvements in hippocampal-dependent memory, synaptic plasticity and cognitive deficits [116, 117]. However, the use of such inhibitors has demonstrated undesirable effects as it may result in acetylation of a range of proteins, thereby creating a target specificity problem [118].

To date, no histone methylation inhibitor compound is used in clinical trials even though therapeutic potential for HD patients. However, there are studies that identified specific inhibitors of methyl transferases (PRC2); these data may be relevant for future research aimed at HD therapy [119].

The following items will also address AMT-130, an artificial miRNA targeting human HTT carried by an AAV5 vector (AAV5-miHTT). Also, the role of Antisense Oligonucleotides (ASO), commonly designed to reduce targeted mutant HTT messenger RNA, will be discussed.

AMT-130

Preclinical data have shown encouraging results for AMT-130 (an uniQure's gene therapy candidate for the treatment of HD) and the U.S. FDA has given fast track designation to it [21]. The designation helps to speed the development, testing, and review of therapies for serious diseases with a high unmet medical need [120]. AMT-130 consists of an AAV5 vector carrying an artificial micro-RNA specifically tailored to silence the HTT gene with the therapeutic goal to inhibit the production of the mHTT protein, the underlying cause of HD [21].

AMT-130 was tested in rodents, mini pigs, and the delivery system tested in nonhuman primates [120, 121, 122]. Of particular interest, significant levels of AMT-130 miRNA were detected in the striatum of mice three months after its injection in this brain area and were accompanied by a marked reduction of the mHTT protein. Further analyses showed improvement in brain cell function and a partial reversal of volume loss in the hippocampus. Besides, no antibodies against AMT-130 were found in cerebrospinal fluid of mini pigs, suggesting that AMT-130's potential is not compromised when administered to the brain or spinal fluid [120].

Using AAV vectors to deliver micro-RNAs directly to the brain for non-selective knockdown of the HTT gene represents a highly innovative and promising approach to treating HD. A planned phase 1/2 trial of the recombinant AAV5 vector treatment is expected briefly to begin dosing patients [21].

Antisense Oligonucleotides (ASO) Targeted to Mutant HTT Messenger RNA

Up to date, a promising approach to deliver effective therapy to HD patients has been developed through gene silencing. Since August 2015, Ionis Pharmaceuticals and several research consortiums [122, 123], have focused efforts designing Antisense Oligonucleotides (ASO) to target specific HTT RNA messenger molecules to inhibit mHTT protein expression, resulting in lower concentration levels of the protein in the cell.

As have been stated earlier, CAG triplet's amplification induces an abnormal protein product that aggregates and accumulates into the cell generating a genotoxic environment and cell death, gliosis and brain atrophy [124, 125]. Even the expression of mutant HTT is not tissue-specific, the major physiopathological feature of HD is displayed in neural tissue leading to degeneration. As a result, HD patients manifest complex CNS diseases including cognitive impairment, neuropsychiatric disturbance and long- and short-term memory dysfunction. For the above-mentioned reasons, research has focused efforts in reducing HTT messenger RNAs in brain tissue, with the aim of improving patient's health conditions, that generally becomes compromised after adulthood. Assuming that the pathology is directly related to the high genotoxic HTT protein levels, researches presume that lowering HTT transcript concentration may improve patients' conditions. In order to test this hypothesis, several clinical trials focus on reducing HTT mRNAs using ASO have been explored. ASO has demonstrated highly effective ability to lower protein expression of HTT, hybridizing to its mRNA and promoting RNase H-induced cleavage of the HTT mRNA.

Although ASOs do not have the capability to cross the blood-brain barrier, their effectiveness has been tested via intrathecal administration. Preclinical data demonstrate that administration of ASO into the cerebrospinal fluid (CSF) delays disease features and phenotype in mice and primate models with no side effects [126, 127]. After intrathecal administration, ASOs spreads throughout the CNS in concordance with the pathology target. For instance, research in primates demonstrates that ASOs accumulates in several brain structures including cortex, hippocampus, pons, cerebellum, spinal cord, and basal ganglia. Moreover, ASOs reduces HTT RNA and HTT protein in a linear proportion to the administrated concentrations. This reduction is more evident in the frontal cortex and spinal cord than in the striatum [127]. Recently, the consortium mentioned above [128] has gone a phase 1/2a clinical trial with an ASO named IONIS-HTTRX, an antisense oligonucleotide designed to inhibit HTT messenger RNA and thereby reduce concentrations of mHTT. The efficacy of IONIS-

HTTRx treatment has resulted in a dose-dependent reduction in the concentration of mHTT in CSF, with a mean of 30% compared to the placebo group.

Based on all the aspects mentioned above, it is emphasized that gene therapy for HD management has increased remarkably over the last years. Despite of many questions that remain in the HD field, ongoing pre-clinical and clinical studies provide a perspective on the mHTT-lowering therapies for HD.

REFERENCES

[1]   Gil-Mohapel, J. M., Rego, A. C. (2011). Huntington's disease: A Review on the Physio pathological Aspects. *Revista Neurociências*, 19 (4): 724-734.

[2]   Kaufmann, K. B., Büning, H., Galy, A., Schambach, A., Grez, M. (2013). Gene therapy on the move. *The EMBO Journal*, 5 (11): 1642-1661.

[3]   Vellai, T., Vida, G. (1999). The origin of eukaryotes: the difference between prokaryotic and eukaryotic cells. *The Royals Society*, 266: 1571-1577.

[4]   Friedmann, T. (1997). The Road toward Human Gene Therapy-A 25-year Perspective. *Annals of Medicine*, 29: 575-577.

[5]   Jackson, D. A., Symons, R. H., Berg, P. (1972). Biochemical Method for Inserting New Genetic Information into DNA of Simian Virus 40: Circular SV40 DNA Molecules Containing Lambda Phage Genes and the Galactose Operon of *Escherichia coli*. *PNAS*, 69 (10): 2904-2909.

[6]   Buckley, R. H. (2004). Molecular Defects in Human Severe Combined Immunodeficiency and Approaches to Immune Reconstitution. *Annual Review of Immunology*, 22: 625-655.

[7]   Schena, M., Shalon, D., Davis, R. W., Brown, P. O. (1995). Quantitative Monitoring of Gene Expression patterns with a Complementary DNA Microarray. *American Association for the Advancement of Science*, 270 (5235): 467-470.

[8]   Mullen, C. A., Snitzer, K., Culver, K. W., Morgan, R. A., Anderson, W. F., Blease, R. M. (1996). Molecular Analysis of T Lymphocyte-Directed Gene Therapy for Adenosine Deaminase Deficiency: Long-Term Expression *In Vivo* of Genes Introduced with a Retroviral Vector. *Human Gene Therapy*, 7 (9): 1123-1129.

[9]   Muul L. M., Tuschong L. M., Soenen S. L., Jagadeesh G. J., Ramsey W. J., Long Z., Carter C. S., Garabedian E. K., Alleyne M., Brown M., Bernstein W., Schurman S. H., Fleisher T. A., Leitman S. F., Dunbar C. E., Blaese R. M., Candotti F. (2003). Persistence and expression of the adenosine deaminase gene for 12 years and immune reaction to gene transfer components: long-term results of the first clinical gene therapy trial. *Blood,* 1;101 (7): 2563-2569.

[10]   Linden, R. (2010). Gene Therapy: what is it, what is not and what will it be. *Estudos avançados* 24 (70).

[11]   Culver, K. W., Osborne, W. R., Miller, A. D., Berger, M., Anderson, W. F., Blaese, R. M. (1991). Correction of ADA deficiency in human T lymphocytes using retroviral-mediated gene transfer. *Transplantation Proceedings*, 23 (1 Pt 1): 170-171.

[12]   Cotrim, A. P., Baum, B. J. (2008). Gene Therapy: Some History, Applications, Problems, and Prospects. *Toxicologic Pathology*, 36 (1): 97-103.

[13]   Choudhury, S. R., Hudry, E., Maguire, C. A., Sena-Esteves, M., Breakefield, X. O., Grandi, P. (2017). Viral vectors for therapy of neurologic diseases. *Neuropharmacology*, 120: 63-80.

[14]   Bardakjian, T. M., Naczi, K. F., Gonzalez-Alegre, P. (2019). Attitudes of Potential Participants towards Molecular Therapy Trials in Huntington's Disease. *Journal Huntingtons Disease*, 8 (1): 79–85.

[15]   Miniarikova, J., Zanella, I., Huseinovic, A., van der Zon, T., Hanemaaijer, E., Martier, R., Koornneef, A., Southwell, A. L., Hayden, M. R., van Deventer, S. J., Petry, H. and Konstantinova, P. (2016). Design, Characterization, and Lead Selection of Therapeutic miRNAs Targeting Huntingtin for Development of Gene Therapy for Huntington's Disease. *Molecular therapy. Nucleic acids*, 5: 297.

[16] Bogdanovic, O., Lister, R. (2017). DNA methylation and the preservation of cell identity. *Current Opinion in Genetics & Development*, 46: 9-14.

[17] Lee, J., Hwang, Y. J., Kim, K. Y., Kowall, N. W. and Ryu, H. (2013). Epigenetic mechanisms of neurodegeneration in Huntington's disease. *Neurotherapeutics,* 10 (4): 664–676.

[18] Moumné, L., Betuing, S. and Caboche, J. (2013). Multiple Aspects of Gene Dysregulation in Huntington's Disease. *Frontiers in Neurology,* 4: 127.

[19] Sharma, S., and Taliyan, R. (2015). Transcriptional dysregulation in Huntington's disease: The role of histone deacetylases. *Pharmacological Research,* 100: 157-169.

[20] Huntington's Disease Society of America (HDSA), (2019). Gene therapy 101. https://hdsa.org/blog/gene-therapy-101/. Accessed July 19.

[21] *uniQure Announces FDA Clearance of Investigational New Drug Application for AMT-130 in Huntington's Disease*, (2019). globenewswire.com/news-release/2019/01/22/1703263/ 0/en/uniQure-Announces-FDA-Clearance-of-Investigational-New-Drug-Application-for-AMT-130-in-Huntington-s-Disease.html. Accessed July 19.

[22] Gene therapy in man. Recommendations of European Medical Research Councils (1998). *The Lancet*, 331: 1271-1272.

[23] Anderson, W. F. (1989). Human Gene Therapy: Why Draw a Line? *The Journal of Medicine and Philosophy*, 14 (6): 681-693.

[24] Rai, S. N., Singh, B. K., Rathore, A. S., Zahra, W., Keswani, C., Birla, H., Singh, S. S., Dilnashin, H., Singh, S. P. (2019). Quality control in huntington's disease: a therapeutic target. *Neurotoxicity Research.* doi: 10.1007/s12640-019-00087-x.

[25] Joshi, A. U., Ebert, A. E., Haileselassie, B., & Mochly-Rosen, D. (2019). Drp1/Fis1-mediated mitochondrial fragmentation leads to lysosomal dysfunction in cardiac models of Huntington's disease. *Journal of Molecular and Cellular Cardiology*, 127: 125–133.

[26]   Martelli, A. (2014). Aspectos clínicos y fisiopatológicos de la enfermedad de Huntington. *Archives of Health Investigation,* 3(4): 32-39. [Clinical and pathophysiological aspects of Huntington's disease. *Archives of Health Investigation,* 3 (4): 32-39].

[27]   Smith-Dijak, A. I., Sepers, M. D. & Raymond, L. A. (2019). Alterations in synaptic function and plasticity in Huntington disease. *Journal of Neurochemistry,* 150 (4): 346-365.

[28]   Cepeda, C., Cummings, D. M., André, V. M., Holley, S. M. and Levine, M. S. (2010). Genetic mouse models of Huntington's disease: focus on electrophysiological mechanisms. *ASN Neuro,* 2 (2), e00033.

[29]   Koch, E. T. and Raymond, L. A. (2019). Dysfunctional striatal dopamine signaling in Huntington's disease. *Journal of Neuroscience Research.* doi: 10.1002/jnr.24495.

[30]   Dvorzhak, A., Helassa, N., Török, K., Schmitz, D. and Grantyn, R. (2019). Single Synapse Indicators of Impaired Glutamate Clearance Derived from Fast iGlu u Imaging of Cortical Afferents in the Striatum of Normal and Huntington (Q175) Mice. *The Journal of Neuroscience,* 39 (20): 3970–3982.

[31]   Boussicault, L., Kacher, R., Lamazière, A., Vanhoutte, P., Caboche, J., Betuing, S. and Potier, M. C. (2018). CYP46A1 protects against NMDA-mediated excitotoxicity in Huntington's disease: Analysis of lipid raft content. *Biochimie,* 153: 70–79.

[32]   Lamirault, C., Yu-Taeger, L., Doyère, V., Riess, O., Nguyen, H. P. and El Massioui, N. (2017). Altered reactivity of central amygdala to GABAAR antagonist in the BACHD rat model of Huntington disease. *Neuropharmacology,* 123: 136–147.

[33]   Hsu, Y. T., Chang, Y. G. and Chern, Y. (2018). Insights into GABAAergic system alteration in Huntington's disease. *Open Biology,* 8 (12): pii: 180165.

[34]   Mattson, M. P. (2006). Neuronal life-and-death signaling, apoptosis, and neurodegenerative disorders. *Antioxidants & Redox Signaling,* 8 (11-12): 1997–2006.

[35]   Intihar, T. A., Martinez, E. A. and Gomez-Pastor, R. (2019). Mitochondrial Dysfunction in Huntington's Disease; Interplay

Between HSF1, p53 and PGC-1α Transcription Factors. *Frontiers in Cellular Neuroscience,* 13: 103.

[36] Tobore, T. O. (2019). Towards a comprehensive understanding of the contributions of mitochondrial dysfunction and oxidative stress in the pathogenesis and pathophysiology of Huntington's disease. *Journal of Neuroscience Research.* doi: 10.1002/jnr.24492.

[37] Stack, E. C. and Ferrante, R. J. (2007). Huntington's disease: progress and potential in the field. *Expert Opinion on Investigational Drugs,* 16 (12): 1933–1953.

[38] Kim, J., Moody, J. P., Edgerly, C. K., Bordiuk, O. L., Cormier, K., Smith, K., Beal, M. F. and Ferrante, R. J. (2010). Mitochondrial loss, dysfunction and altered dynamics in Huntington's disease. *Human Molecular Genetics,* 19 (20): 3919–3935.

[39] Damiano, M., Galvan, L., Déglon, N. and Brouillet, E. (2010). Mitochondria in Huntington's disease. *Biochimica et Biophysica Acta,* 1802 (1): 52–61.

[40] Kumar, A. and Ratan, R. R. (2016). Oxidative stress and huntington's disease: the good, the bad, and the ugly. *Journal of Huntington's Disease,* 5 (3): 217–237.

[41] Dufour, B. D., Smith, C. A., Clark, R. L., Walker, T. R. and McBride, J. L. (2014). Intrajugular vein delivery of AAV9-RNAi prevents neuropathological changes and weight loss in Huntington's disease mice. *Molecular Therapy,* 22 (4): 797–810.

[42] Stanek, L. M., Bu, J. and Shihabuddin, L. S. (2019). Astrocyte transduction is required for rescue of behavioral phenotypes in the YAC128 mouse model with AAV-RNAi mediated HTT lowering therapeutics. *Neurobiology of Disease,* 129: 29–37.

[43] Bradford, J., Shin, J. Y., Roberts, M., Wang, C. E., Li, X. J. and Li, S. (2009). Expression of mutant huntingtin in mouse brain astrocytes causes age-dependent neurological symptoms. *Proceedings of the National Academy of Sciences of the United States of America,* 106 (52): 22480–22485.

[44]   Goodall, E. F., Heath, P. R., Bandmann, O., Kirby, J., and Shaw, P. J. (2013). Neuronal dark matter: the emerging role of microRNAs in neurodegeneration. *Frontiers in Cellular Neuroscience,* 7: 178.

[45]   Lau, P., and de Strooper, B. (2010). Dysregulated microRNAs in neurodegenerative disorders. *Seminars in Cell & Developmental Biology,* 21: 768–773.

[46]   Yin, S., Yu, Y., and Reed, R. (2015). Primary microRNA processing is functionally coupled to RNAP II transcription in vitro. *Scientific Reports,* 5: 11992.

[47]   Winter, J., Jung, S., Keller, S., Gregory, R. I., and Diederichs, S. (2009). Many roads to maturity: microRNA biogenesis pathways and their regulation. *Nature Cell Biology,* 11: 228–234.

[48]   Rupaimoole, R., Slack, F. J. (2017). MicroRNA therapeutics: towards a new era for the management of cancer and other diseases. *Nature Reviews; Drug Discovery,* 16 (3): 203-222.

[49]   Martí, E., Pantano, L., Bañez-Coronel, M., Llorens, F., Miñones-Moyano, E., Porta, S., Sumoy L., Ferrer I., Estivill X. (2010). A myriad of miRNA variants in control and Huntington's disease brain regions detected by massively parallel sequencing. *Nucleic Acids Research,* 38: 7219–7235.

[50]   Zuccato, C., Tartari, M., Crotti, A., Goffredo, D., Valenza, M., Conti, L., Cataudella, T., Leavitt, B. R., Hayden, M. R., Timmusk, T., Rigamonti, D., Cattaneo, E. (2003). Huntingtin interacts with REST/NRSF to modulate the transcription of NRSE-controlled neuronal genes. *Nature Genetics,* 35: 76 –83.

[51]   Andre´s, M. E., Burger, C., Peral-Rubio, M. J., Battaglioli, E., Anderson, M. E., Grimes, J., Dallman, J., Ballas, N., Mandel, G. (1999). CoREST: a functional corepressor required for regulation of neural-specific gene expression. *Proceedings of the National Academy of Science of the USA*, 96: 9873–9878.

[52]   Conaco, C., Otto, S., Han, J. J., Mandel, G. (2006). Reciprocal actions of REST and a microRNA promote neuronal identity. *Proceedings of the National Academy of Science of the USA*, 103: 2422–2427.

[53] Zuccato, C., Belyaev, N., Conforti, P., Ooi, L., Tartari, M., Papadimou, E., MacDonald, M., Fossale, E., Zeitlin, S., Buckley, N. and Cattaneo, E. (2007). Widespread disruption of repressor element-1 silencing transcription factor/neuron-restrictive silencer factor occupancy at its target genes in Huntington's disease. *The Journal of Neuroscience,* 27 (26): 6972–6983.

[54] Packer, A. N., Xing, Y., Harper, S. Q., Jones, L., & Davidson, B. L. (2008). The Bifunctional microRNA miR-9/miR-9* Regulates REST and CoREST and Is Downregulated in Huntington's Disease. *Journal of Neuroscience,* 28 (53): 14341–14346.

[55] Vo, N., Klein, M. E., Varlamova, O., Keller, D. M., Yamamoto, T., Goodman, R. H., Impey, S. (2005). A cAMP-response element binding protein-induced microRNA regulates neuronal morpho-genesis. *Proceedings of the National Academy of Science of the USA,* 102: 16426 –16431.

[56] Mortazavi, A., Thompson, E. C. L., Garcia, S. T., Myers, R. M., Wold, B. (2006) Comparative genomics modeling of the NRSF/REST repressor network: from single conserved sites to genome-wide repertoire. *Genome Research,* 16: 1208 –1221.

[57] Lim, L. P., Lau, N. C., Garrett-Engele, P., Grimson, A., Schelter, J. M., Castle, J., Bartel, D. P., Linsley, P. S., Johnson, J. M. (2005). Microarray analysis shows that some microRNAs downregulate large numbers of target mRNAs. *Nature,* 433: 769 –773.

[58] Akerblom, M., Sachdeva, R., Barde, I., Verp, S., Gentner, B., Trono, D., Jakobsson, J. (2012). MicroRNA-124 is a subventricular zone neuronal fate determinant. *The Journal of Neuroscience,* 32: 8879-8889.

[59] Hodges, A., Strand, A. D., Aragaki, A. K., Kuhn, A., Sengstag, T., Hughes, G., Elliston, L. A., Hartog, C., Goldstein, D. R., Thu, D., Hollingsworth, Z. R., Collin, F., Synek, B., Holmans, P. A., Young, A. B., Wexler, N. S., Delorenzi, M., Kooperberg, C., Augood, S. J., Faull, R. L., Olson, J. M., Jones, L., Luthi-Carter, R. (2006). Regional and cellular gene expression changes in human Huntington's disease brain. *Human Molecular Genetics,* 15: 965–977.

[60]   Zuccato, C., Ciammola, A., Rigamonti, D., Leavitt, B. R., Goffredo, D., Conti, L., MacDonald, M. E., Friedlander, R. M., Silani, V., Hayden, M. R., Timmusk, T., Sipione, S., Cattaneo, E. (2001). Loss of huntingtin-mediated BDNF gene transcription in Huntington's disease. *Science,* 293: 493-498.

[61]   Zuccato, C., & Cattaneo, E. (2007). Role of brain-derived neurotrophic factor in Huntington's disease. *Progress in Neurobiology,* 81 (5-6): 294–330.

[62]   Zuccato, C., Marullo, M., Vitali, B., Tarditi, A., Mariotti, C., Valenza, M., Lahiri, N., Wild, E. J., Sassone, J., Ciammola, A., Bachoud-Levi, A. C., Tabrizi, S. J., Di Donato, S., Cattaneo, E. (2011). Brain-derived neurotrophic factor in patients with Huntington's disease. *PLoS One* 6: e22966.

[63]   Ciammola, A., Sassone, J., Cannella, M., Calza, S., Poletti, B., Frati, L., Squitieri, F., Silani, V. (2007). Low brain-derived neurotrophic factor (BDNF) levels in serum of Huntington's disease patients. *American Journal of Medical Genetics, Part B, Neuropsychiatric Genetics,* 144B (4): 574-577.

[64]   Strand, A. D., Baquet, Z. C., Aragaki, A. K., Holmans, P., Yang, L., Cleren, C., Beal, M. F., Jones, L., Kooperberg, C., Olson, J. M., Jones, K. R. (2007). Expression profiling of Huntington's disease models suggests that brain-derived neurotrophic factor depletion plays a major role in striatal degeneration. *The Journal of Neuroscience,* 27: 11758-11768.

[65]   Tian, L., Wooseok, I., Inhee, M. J., Manho, K. (2015). MicroRNA-124 slows down the progression of Huntington's disease by promoting neurogenesis in the striatum. *Neural Regeneration Research,* 10: 786-791.

[66]   Klein, M. E., Lioy, D. T., Ma, L., Impey, S., Mandel, G., Goodman, R. H. (2007). Homeostatic regulation of MeCP2 expression by a CREB-induced microRNA. *Nature Neuroscience,* 10: 1513–1514.

[67]   Lunyak, V. V., Burgess, R., Prefontaine, G. G., Nelson, C., Sze, S. H., Chenoweth, J., Schwartz, P., Pevzner, P. A., Glass, C., Mandel, G., Rosenfeld, M. G. (2002). Corepressor-dependent silencing of

chromosomal regions encoding neuronal genes. *Science,* 298: 1747–1752.

[68] Fukuoka, M., Takahashi, M., Fujita, H., Chiyo, T., Popiel, H. A., Watanabe, S., Furuya, H., Murata, M., Wada, K., Okada, T., Nagai, Y., Hohjoh, H. (2018). Supplemental treatment for Huntington 's disease with mir-132 that is deficient in Huntington's disease brain. *Molecular Therapy; Nucleic Acids,* 11: 79–90.

[69] Johnson, R., Zuccato, C., Belyaev, N. D., Guest, D. J., Cattaneo, E., and Buckley, N. J. (2008). A microRNA-based gene dysregulation pathway in Huntington's disease. *Neurobiology of Diseases*, 29: 438–445.

[70] Jovicic, A., Zaldivar Jolissaint, J. F., Moser, R., Silva Santos, M. de F., & Luthi-Carter, R. (2013). MicroRNA-22 (miR-22) Overexpression Is Neuroprotective via General Anti-Apoptotic Effects and May also Target Specific Huntington's Disease-Related Mechanisms. *PLoS ONE,* 8 (1): e54222.

[71] Yin, H., Kanasty, R. L., Eltoukhy, A. A., Vegas, A. J., Dorkin, J. R. and Anderson, D. G. (2014). Non-viral vectors for gene-based therapy. *Nature Reviews. Genetics,* 15 (8):541–555.

[72] Qu Y., Liu Y., Noor A. F., Tran J., Li R. (2019). Characteristics and advantages of adeno-associated virus vector-mediated gene therapy for neurodegenerative diseases. *Neural Regeneration Research*, 14 (6): 931–938.

[73] Lundstrom, K. (2018). Viral Vectors in Gene Therapy. *Diseases,* 6 (2): 42.

[74] Chira, S., Jackson, C. S., Oprea, I., Ozturk, F., Pepper, M. S., Diaconu, I., Braicu, C., Raduly, L. Z., Calin, G. A., Berindan-Neagoe, I. (2015). Progresses towards safe and efficient gene therapy vectors. *Oncotarget*, 6 (31): 30675-30703.

[75] Coura, R. (2012). Viral vectors in neurobiology: therapeutic and research applications. In: Adoga, M. P., editor. *Molecular virology* Shanghai: InTech 5: 75-93.

[76] Chun, H., Marriott, I., Lee, C. J. and Cho, H. (2018). Elucidating the interactive roles of glia in Alzheimer 's disease using established and

newly developed experimental models. *Frontiers in Neurology,* 9: 797.

[77]   Vagner, T., Dvorzhak, A., Wójtowicz, A. M., Harms, C. and Grantyn, R. (2016). Systemic application of AAV vectors targeting GFAP-expressing astrocytes in Z-Q175-KI Huntington's disease mice. *Molecular and Cellular Neurosciences,* 7776–7786.

[78]   Lee, J., Hwang, Y. J., Shin, J. Y., Lee, W. C., Wie, J., Kim, K. Y., Lee, M. Y., Hwang, D., Ratan, R. R., Pae, A. N., Kowall, N. W., So, I., Kim, J. I. and Ryu, H. (2013). Epigenetic regulation of cholinergic receptor M1 (CHRM1) by histone H3K9me3 impairs Ca(2+) signaling in Huntington's disease. *Acta Neuropathologica,* 125 (5): 727–739.

[79]   Thomas, E. A. (2016). DNA methylation in Huntington's disease: Implications for transgenerational effects. *Neuroscience Letters,* 625: 34–39.

[80]   Razin, A. and Riggs, A. D. (1980). DNA methylation and gene function. *Science,* 210(4470): 604–610.

[81]   Breiling, A. and Lyko, F. (2015). Epigenetic regulatory functions of DNA modifications: 5-methylcytosine and beyond. *Epigenetics & Chromatin,* 8: 24.

[82]   Chahrour, M. and Zoghbi, H. Y. (2007). The story of Rett syndrome: from clinic to neurobiology. *Neuron,* 56 (3): 422–437.

[83]   Goll, M. G., Kirpekar, F., Maggert, K. A., Yoder, J. A., Hsieh, C.-L., Zhang, X., Golic, K. G., Jacobsen, S. E. and Bestor, T. H. (2006). Methylation of tRNAAsp by the DNA methyltransferase homolog Dnmt2. *Science,* 311 (5759): 395–398.

[84]   Moore, L. D., Le, T. and Fan, G. (2013). DNA Methylation and Its Basic Function. *Neuropsychopharmacology,* 38 (1): 23-38.

[85]   Klein, C. J., Botuyan, M. V., Wu, Y., Ward, C. J., Nicholson, G. A., Hammans, S., Hojo, K., Yamanishi, H., Karpf, A. R., Wallace, D. C., Simon, M., Lander, C., Boardman, L. A., Cunningham, J. M., Smith, G. E., Litchy, W. J., Boes, B., Atkinson, E. J., Middha, S., B Dyck, P. J., Parisi, J. E., Mer, G., Smith, D. I. and Dyck, P. J. (2011). Mutations

in DNMT1 cause hereditary sensory neuropathy with dementia and hearing loss. *Nature Genetics,* 43 (6): 595–600.

[86] Watt, F. and Molloy, P. L. (1988). Cytosine methylation prevents binding to DNA of a HeLa cell transcription factor required for optimal expression of the adenovirus major late promoter. *Genes & Development,* 2 (9): 1136–1143.

[87] Bird, A. P. (1986). CpG-rich islands and the function of DNA methylation. *Nature,* 321 (6067): 209-213.

[88] Ng, C. W., Yildirim, F., Yap, Y. S., Dalin, S., Matthews, B. J., Velez, P. J., Labadorf, A., Housman, D. E. and Fraenkel, E. (2013). Extensive changes in DNA methylation are associated with expression of mutant huntingtin. *Proceedings of the National Academy of Sciences of the USA,* 110 (6): 2354–2359.

[89] Wood, H. (2013). Neurodegenerative disease: altered DNA methylation and RNA splicing could be key mechanisms in Huntington disease. *Nature Reviews. Neurology,* 9 (3): 119.

[90] Gil, J. M. and Rego, A. C. (2008). Mechanisms of neurodegeneration in Huntington's disease. *The European Journal of Neuroscience,* 27 (11): 2803–2820.

[91] Kerschbamer, E. and Biagioli, M. (2015). Huntington's Disease as Neurodevelopmental Disorder: Altered Chromatin Regulation, Coding, and Non-Coding RNA Transcription. *Frontiers in Neuroscience,* 9: 509.

[92] Jia, H., Morris, C. D., Williams, R. M., Loring, J. F. and Thomas, E. A. (2015). HDAC inhibition imparts beneficial transgenerational effects in Huntington's disease mice via altered DNA and histone methylation. *Proceedings of the National Academy of Sciences of the USA,* 112 (1): 56–64.

[93] Introduction to Glutamine repeats and neurodegenerative diseases: molecular aspects. A Discussion Meeting held at the Royal Society on 7 and 8 October 1998. (1999). *Philosophical Transactions of the Royal Society B: Biological Sciences,* 354 (1386): 957–961.

[94] Reiner, A., Albin, R. L., Anderson, K. D., D'Amato, C. J., Penney, J. B. and Young, A. B. (1988). Differential loss of striatal projection

neurons in Huntington disease. *Proceedings of the National Academy of Sciences of the USA,* 85 (15): 5733–5737.

[95]   Villar-Menéndez, I., Blanch, M., Tyebji, S., Pereira-Veiga, T., Albasanz, J. L., Martín, M., Ferrer, I., Pérez-Navarro, E., Barrachina, M. (2013). Increased 5-methylcytosine and decreased 5-hydroxymethylcytosine levels are associated with reduced striatal A2AR levels in Huntington's disease. *Neuromolecular Medicine,* 15 (2): 295-309.

[96]   Zuccato, C., Marullo, M., Conforti, P., MacDonald, M. E., Tartari, M. and Cattaneo, E. (2008). Systematic assessment of BDNF and its receptor levels in human cortices affected by Huntington's disease. *Brain Pathology,* 18 (2): 225–238.

[97]   Tebano, M. T., Martire, A., Chiodi, V., Ferrante, A. and Popoli, P. (2010). Role of adenosine A(2A) receptors in modulating synaptic functions and brain levels of BDNF: a possible key mechanism in the pathophysiology of Huntington's disease. *The Scientific World Journal,* 10: 1768–1782.

[98]   Thomas, B., Matson, S., Chopra, V., Sun, L., Sharma, S., Hersch, S., Rosas, H. D., Scherzer, C., Ferrante, R. and Matson, W. (2013). A novel method for detecting 7-methyl guanine reveals aberrant methylation levels in Huntington disease. *Analytical Biochemistry,* 436 (2): 112–120.

[99]   Sadri-Vakili, G. and Cha, J. H. J. (2006). Mechanisms of disease: Histone modifications in Huntington's disease. Nature Clinical Practice. *Neurology,* 2 (6): 330–338.

[100] Jenuwein, T. and Allis, C. D. (2001). Translating the histone code. *Science,* 293 (5532): 1074–1080.

[101] Bassi, S., Tripathi, T., Monziani, A., Di Leva, F. and Biagioli, M. (2017). Epigenetics of Huntington's disease. *Advances in Experimental Medicine and Biology,* 978: 277–299.

[102] Ganai, S., Banday, S., Farooq, Z., Altaf, M. (2016). Modulating epigenetic HAT activity for reinstating acetylation homeostasis: A promising therapeutic strategy for neurological disorders. *Pharmacology & Therapeutics,* 166: 106-22.

[103] Galvan, L., Francelle, L., Gaillard, M. C., de Longprez, L., Carrillo-de Sauvage, M. A., Liot, G., Cambon, K., Stimmer, L., Luccantoni, S., Flament, J., Valette, J., de Chaldée, M., Auregan, G., Guillermier, M., Joséphine, C., Petit, F., Jan, C., Jarrige, M., Dufour, N., Bonvento, G., Humbert, S., Saudou, F., Hantraye, P., Merienne, K., Bemelmans, A. P., Perrier, A. L., Déglon, N. and Brouillet, E. (2018). The striatal kinase DCLK3 produces neuroprotection against mutant huntingtin. *Brain: A Journal of Neurology,* 141 (5): 1434–1454.

[104] Bates, E. A., Victor, M., Jones, A. K., Shi, Y., Hart, A. C. (2006). Differential contributions of Caenorhabditis elegans histone deacetylases to huntingtin polyglutamine toxicity. *Journal of Neuroscience*, 26: 2830–2838.

[105] Dompierre, J. P., Godin, J. D., Charrin, B. C., Cordelières, F. P., King, S. J., Humbert, S., Saudou, F. (2007). Histone deacetylase 6 inhibition compensates for the transport deficit in Huntington's disease by increasing tubulin acetylation. *Journal of Neuroscience,* 27: 3571–3583.

[106] McCampbell, A., Taye, A. A., Whitty, L., Penney, E., Steffan, J. S. and Fischbeck, K. H. (2001). Histone deacetylase inhibitors reduce polyglutamine toxicity. *Proceedings of the National Academy of Sciences of the USA,* 98 (26): 15179–15184.

[107] Steffan, J. S., Bodai, L., Pallos, J., Poelman, M., McCampbell, A., Apostol, B. L., Kazantsev, A., Schmidt, E., Zhu, Y. Z., Greenwald, M., Kurokawa, R., Housman, D. E., Jackson, G. R., Marsh, J. L. and Thompson, L. M. (2001). Histone deacetylase inhibitors arrest polyglutamine-dependent neurodegeneration in Drosophila. *Nature,* 413 (6857): 739–743.

[108] Hughes, R. E., Lo, R. S., Davis, C., Strand, A. D., Neal, C. L., Olson, J. M. and Fields, S. (2001). Altered transcription in yeast expressing expanded polyglutamine. *Proceedings of the National Academy of Sciences of the USA,* 98(23): 13201–13206.

[109] Perutz, M. F., Johnson, T., Suzuki, M. and Finch, J. T. (1994). Glutamine repeats as polar zippers: their possible role in inherited

neurodegenerative diseases. *Proceedings of the National Academy of Sciences of the USA,* 91(12): 5355–5358.

[110] Cha, J. H. (2000). Transcriptional dysregulation in Huntington's disease. *Trends in Neurosciences,* 23 (9): 387–392.

[111] Greer, E. L., Shi, Y. (2012). Histone methylation: a dynamic mark in health, disease and inheritance. *Nature Reviews. Genetics,* 13 (5): 343-57.

[112] Maes, T., Mascaró, C., Ortega, A., Lunardi, S., Ciceri, F., Somervaille, T. C. P. and Buesa, C. (2015). KDM1 histone lysine demethylases as targets for treatments of oncological and neurodegenerative disease. *Epigenomics,* 7(4): 609–626.

[113] Song, W., Zsindely, N., Faragó, A., Marsh, J. L. and Bodai, L. (2018). Systematic genetic interaction studies identify histone demethylase Utx as potential target for ameliorating Huntington's disease. *Human Molecular Genetics,* 27 (4): 649–666.

[114] Ryu, H., Lee, J., Hagerty, S. W., Soh, B. Y., McAlpin, S. E., Cormier, K. A., Smith, K. M. and Ferrante, R. J. (2006). ESET/SETDB1 gene expression and histone H3 (K9) trimethylation in Huntington's disease. *Proceedings of the National Academy of Sciences of the United States of America,* 103 (50): 19176–19181.

[115] Ratovitski, T., Arbez, N., Stewart, J. C., Chighladze, E. and Ross, C. A. (2015). PRMT5- mediated symmetric arginine dimethylation is attenuated by mutant huntingtin and is impaired in Huntington's disease (HD). *Cell Cycle,* 14 (11): 1716–1729.

[116] Hogarth, P., Lovrecic, L. and Krainc, D. (2007). Sodium phenylbutyrate in Huntington's disease: a dose-finding study. *Movement Disorders,* 22 (13): 1962–1964.

[117] Lopez-Atalaya, J. P., Ito, S., Valor, L. M., Benito, E. and Barco, A. (2013). Genomic targets, and histone acetylation and gene expression profiling of neural HDAC inhibition. *Nucleic Acids Research,* 41 (17): 8072–8084.

[118] Choudhary, C., Kumar, C., Gnad, F., Nielsen, M. L., Rehman, M., Walther, T. C., Olsen, J. V. and Mann, M. (2009). Lysine acetylation

targets protein complexes and co-regulates major cellular functions. *Science*, 325 (5942): 834–840.

[119] McCabe, M. T., Ott, H. M., Ganji, G., Korenchuk, S., Thompson, C., Aller, G. S. V., Liu, Y., Graves, A. P., Pietra III, A. D., Diaz, E., LaFrance, L. V., Mellinger, M., Duquenne, C., Tian, X., Kruger, R. G., McHugh, C. F., Brandt, M., Miller, W. H., Dhanak, D., Verma, S. K., Tummino, P. J., Creasy, C. L., (2012). EZH2 inhibition as a therapeutic strategy for lymphoma with EZH2-activating mutations. *Nature,* 492 (7427): 108–112.

[120] *Huntington's Disease News.* (2019). FDA Places Gene Therapy AMT-130 on Fast Track to Speed Development. https://huntington sdiseasenews.com/2019/04/11/fda-places-gene-therapy-amt-130-on-fast-track-to-speed-development/. Acessed august 19.

[121] uniQure's. (2019). *uniQure has submitted an IND and is posed to become the first gene therapy to enter the clinic in Huntington's disease.* http://uniqure.com/gene-therapy/huntingtons-disease.php. Acessed august 19.

[122] Potkin, K. T. and Potkin, S. G. (2018). New directions in therapeutics for Huntington disease. *Future neurology,* 13 (2): 101–121.

[123] Hays P. (2016). *Meet the compound: IONIS-HTTRx.* HD Insights 13: 13.

[124] Rollnik, J. D. (2017). Hope for Huntington's disease patients: first clinical gene silencing study in progress. *Fortschritte der Neurologie-Psychiatrie,* 85 (8): 463–466.

[125] Vonsattel, J. P., Myers, R. H., Stevens, T. J., Ferrante, R. J., Bird, E. D. and Richardson, E. P. (1985). Neuropathological classification of Huntington's disease. *Journal of Neuropathology and Experimental Neurology,* 44 (6): 559–577.

[126] Lane, R. M., Smith, A., Baumann, T., Gleichmann, M., Norris, D., Bennett, C. F. and Kordasiewicz, H. (2018). Translating Antisense Technology into a Treatment for Huntington's Disease. *Methods in Molecular Biology,* 1780: 497–523.

[127] Kordasiewicz, H. B., Stanek, L. M., Wancewicz, E. V., Mazur, C., McAlonis, M. M., Pytel, K. A., Artates, J. W., Weiss, A., Cheng, S.

H., Shihabuddin, L. S., Hung, G., Bennett, C. F., Cleveland, D. W. (2012). Sustained therapeutic reversal of Huntington's disease by transient repression of huntingtin synthesis. *Neuron,* 74: 1031–1044.

[128] Van Roon-Mom, W. M. C., Roos, R. A. C. and de Bot, S. T. (2018). Dose-Dependent Lowering of Mutant Huntingtin Using Antisense Oligonucleotides in Huntington Disease Patients. *Nucleic acid therapeutics,* 28 (2): 59–62.

[129] Tabrizi, S. J., Leavitt, B. R., Landwehrmeyer, G. B., Wild, E. J., Saft, C., Barker, R. A., Blair, N. F., Craufurd, D., Priller, J., Rickards, H., Rosser, A., Kordasiewicz, H. B., Czech, C., Swayze, E. E., Norris, D. A., Baumann, T., Gerlach, I., Schobel, S. A., Paz, E., Smith, A. V., Bennett, C. F. and Lane, R. M. (2019). Targeting Huntingtin Expression in Patients with Huntington's Disease. *The New England Journal of Medicine,* 380 (24): 2307–2316.

INDEX

Q

R

S

T

V

W

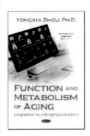
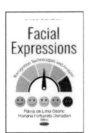

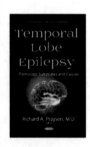